Systematic Medical Terminology

By

Dr. Mohammed Bin Abdullah Bin Ali Alqumber
Associate Professor of Medical Laboratory Medicine
and Medical Microbiology
Faculty of Applied Medical Sciences
Albaha University
Saudi Arabia

Print information available on the last page.

Rev. date: 03/26/2015

To order additional copies of this book, contact:
Xlibris
1663 Liberty Drive
Suite 200
Bloomington IN 47403
1-800-455-039
www.xlibris.com.au
Orders@Xlibris.com.au

Systematic Medical Terminology

By

Dr. Mohammed Bin Abdullah Bin Ali Alqumber
Associate Professor of Medical Laboratory Medicine
and Medical Microbiology
Faculty of Applied Medical Sciences
Albaha University
Saudi Arabia

Acknowledgments

This book is a direct result of encouragement from the Governor of Albaha Province His Royal Highness Price Mishary Bin Saud & His Excellency the Rector of Albaha University Professor Saad Alhareky. Both kept their hearts & quarters open for my reception & regularly motivated, encouraged & nurtured contributions to science. Also, this book would not be possible if it were not for the support from my great Wife. Finally, I must acknowledge my Father for his indispensable & continuous support & wise advise.

Dedication

To His Majesty King Abdullah Bin Abdulaziz.

The Custodian of The Two Holy Mosques.

To His Royal Highness Price Mishary Bin Saud Bin Abdulaziz.

The Governor of Albaha Province.

To His Excellency Professor Saad Bin Mohammed Alhareky.

The Rector of Albaha University.

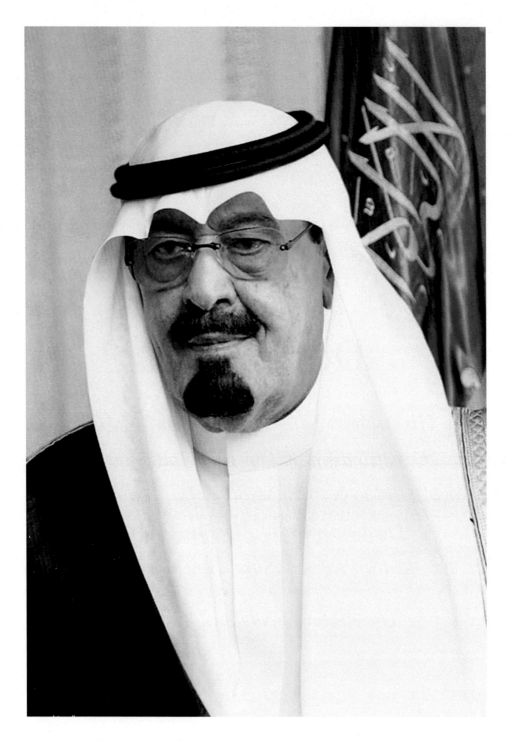

His Majesty King Abdullah Bin Abdulaziz.

The Custodian of the Two Holy Mosques

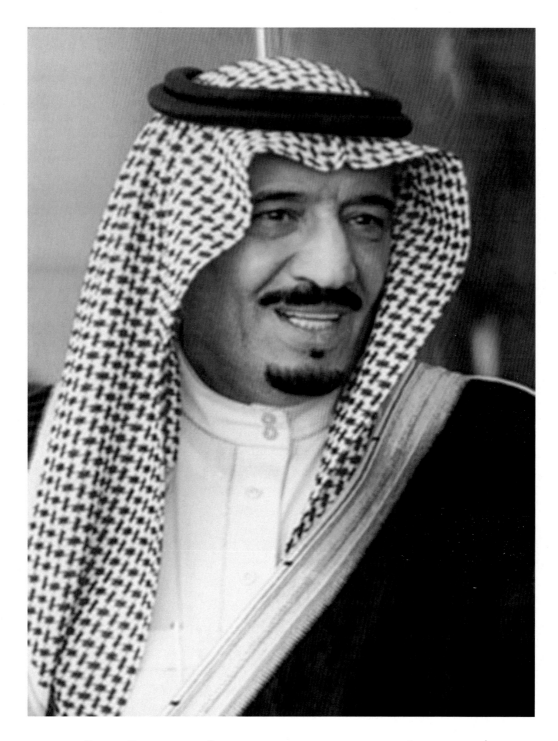

His Majesty King Salman Bin Abdulaziz.

The Custodian of the Two Holy Mosques

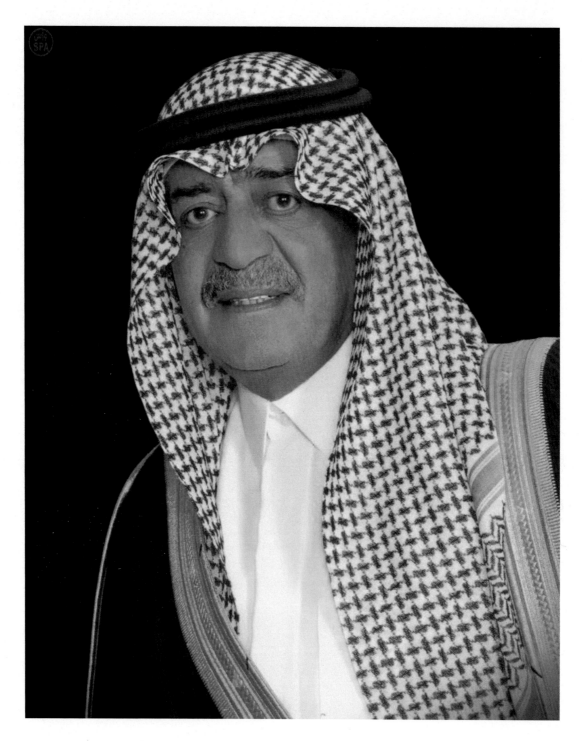

His Royal Highness Prince Muqrin Bin Abdulaziz,

Crown Prince

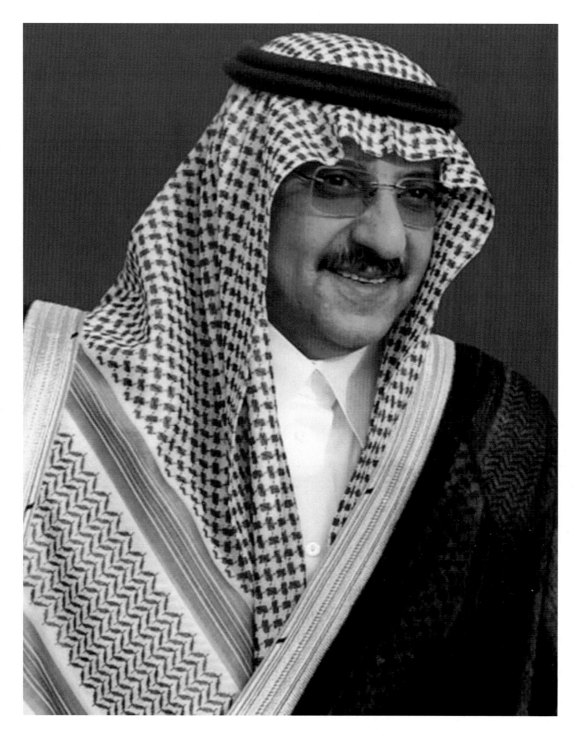

His Royal Highness Prince Mohammed Bin Naif Bin

Deputy Crown Prince

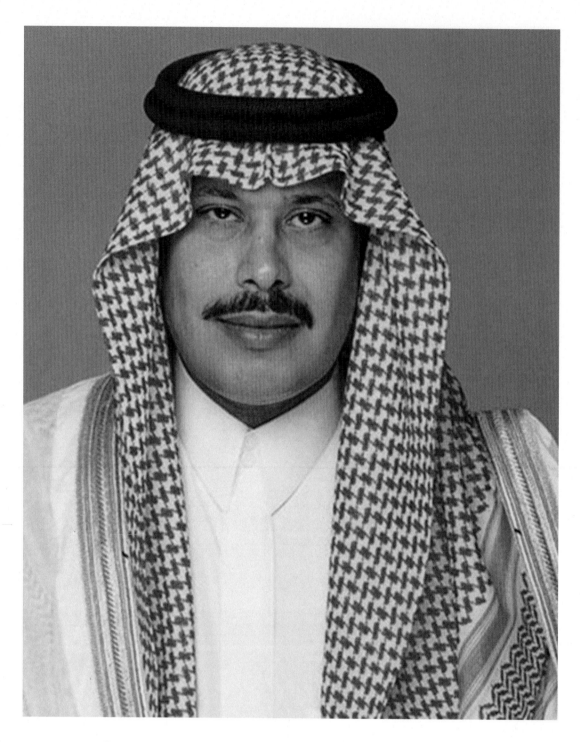

His Royal Highness Prince Mishary Bin Saud Bin Abdulaziz.

The Governor of Albaha Province

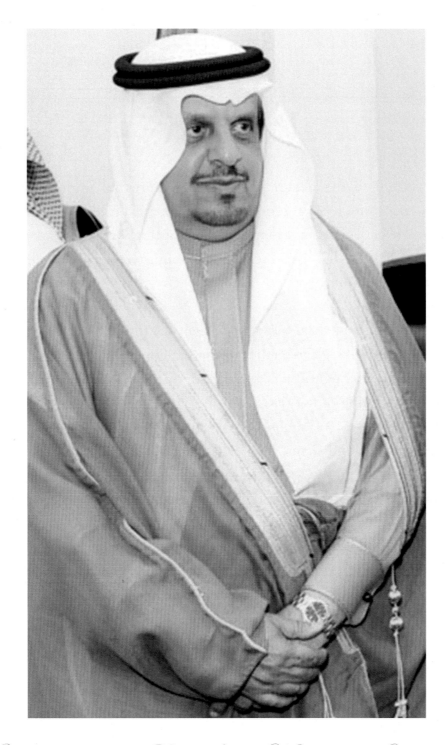

His Excellency Prof. Saad Mohammed Alhareky

President of Albaha University

Preface

Everyone related to the health professions requires an understanding of medical terminology. Students must have a good command of medical terminology to be able to understand medical texts. That is, in order to read medical reports and books, complete forms, and communicate with others in the medical field, one must have a good understanding of the principles of medical terminology.

At the first instance, medical terms may seem confusing and difficult to understand. Fortunately, however, there is logic to medical terms that, once grasped, can help make it much easier to understand them. Medical terms are made of parts, each with a defined meaning. Once you know the meaning of the parts you can figure the meaning of the whole medical term. These parts are identified as stems, prefixes and suffixes. Many medical terms will share the same prefixes, suffixes and stems; they can hence be used in different combinations to mean different things. Herein you will learn to identify these parts and how they can be used in different combinations to construct and describe medical terms and conditions.

This book is intended for students studying medical disciplines, such as medicine, dentistry, laboratory medicine, nursing, physiotherapy, community health, preventative medicine, radiology and clinical nutrition. It will help the reader understand the basic language of medicine. It is written as a comprehensive systematic framework classifying, defining and tabulating medical terms, and can therefore be used as a useful resource and reference. Its final goal is to help you understand and convert any medical term into lay language; thus, when you are you given the medical term, you will be able to identify the proper definition, or when given the definition of a medical term you will be able to construct and identify the proper medical term.

Contents

CHAPTER 1

BASIC COMPONENTS

Chapter Contents

PART 1:1 MEDICAL ENGLISH – HOW AND WHY TO LEARN IT

The names of bodily organs, tissues, diseases, and treatments are best communicated in medical English. ***Learning medical English is an obligation in the medical profession since no language other than English covers all the new discoveries in detail and in a timely fashion.*** This is because English is today's international language of communication between scientists. However, comprehending medical English has traditionally been one of the most serious disadvantages of heath care students from non-English-speaking countries. Therefore, this book is written to provide a practical approach for the learning of medical English to non-English speaking students. In conjunction with this manual, you should regularly read professional medical manuscripts. Reading professional manuscripts is the best way to inform oneself and to learn, and since the medical field is constantly changing, one must be reading constantly to remain up to date, otherwise the safety and health of involved patients would be endangered. While it is difficult to read medical English out loud at the beginning because many words are very difficult to pronounce, even when you may already know their meaning and spelling, it is important to do so: reading words out loud will improve your learning results three times over by making the reading exercise a reading, listening and speaking exercise. I would encourage you to do this from the start of your learning journey. Moreover, reading out loud will prevent poor pronunciation, which leads to low self-confidence and poor communication.

Also, try always to write down each new medical term on a scrap piece of paper or in a notebook a number of times. This will help you memorize them and retain their structure, meaning and spelling. Finally, remember that satisfactory data retention can be aided by *spaced repetition* and *mnemonic techniques*. **Space repetition is a learning technique where the information studied is reviewed subsequently at increasing intervals of time to increase the retention of information**. Basically, you need to review information repeatedly to remember it for a considerable time, but the time between repeats must grow exponentially longer after each repeat for optimal success. Repeat something too early and you waste time, repeat it too late and you have forgotten it and may have to relearn it from the very beginning as if you had not heard of it before. This will lead you to waste your time and energy. The ideal repetition time is before you forget 50% of the information you learned. The spaced repetition technique states that if you have a piece of information you need to memorize in a limited time (because you have other subjects to learn and a other activities), then the best way is to divide the available time into spaced repeats as Figure 1 illustrates.

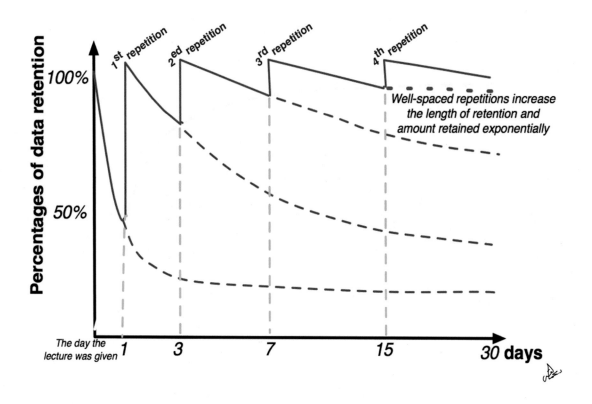

Figure 1: Illustration of the spaced repetition technique.

Mnemonic techniques are memorization methods that aid information retention without repetition through the translation of information into a form that the human brain can retain. Common mnemonic techniques are used to memorize lists and link causes and effects. Mnemonic techniques include poems, acronyms, phrases and visual aids. For example, since the only transparent renal stones in radiology films (radiolucent stones) are <u>u</u>ric acid stones, a possible mnemonic technique to remember this fact can be the following: think "<u>U</u>" of "uric acid" equals "<u>U</u>" of "<u>u</u>nseen in radiographs."

PART 1:2 THE PLURAL AND SINGULAR FORMS OF MEDICAL NOUNS

Specialized medical terminology consists mainly of Latin and Greek words. Many of these words have retained the rule for the formation of the plural from their original language, and you thus need to know how to pluralize Latin and Greek nouns as part of your medical education.

Latin has three types of nouns, plus some exceptions. Latin nouns can take one of various forms, which are called "declensions." The declension of a noun depends on how it is gendered – that is, masculine, feminine, or neuter – but this arrangement is largely arbitrary and you do not need to try and understand the basis of it. Nonetheless, it does explain the reasons for the observed differences in pluralizing them. What you need to remember is that nouns ending in -a (feminine nouns) are pluralized by making the noun end with -ae; nouns ending with -us (masculine nouns) are pluralized by changing the ending to -i; and nouns ending in -um (neuter nouns) are pluralized by changing the ending to -a. For example, "antenna" becomes "antennae," "focus" becomes "foci," and "medium" becomes "media." Table 1 lists more examples. These are easy to grasp, but there are some exceptions. Most of these exceptions will have a plural form ending with -es. Examples of such nouns include ones ending with "-is"; you can just remove the "-is" and add "-es" on to the end of the noun to make it plural. For example, the word crisis is pluralized as crises, thesis as theses, axis as axes, and diagnosis as diagnoses. Other exceptions include nouns like the word "index," whose root is "indic" and whose plural form is "indices." Similarly, nouns like appendix, matrix and thorax are pluralized appendices, matrices and thoraces, respectively. Now, we will introduce to you the Greek nouns ending with "-ma." These nouns are pluralized by making them end with "-mata." For example, stoma will become stomata (Table 1). Finally, an important exception to the above is the noun "genus." This is not a "simple" second-declension masculine noun, as it appears, but a third-declension neuter noun; its plural is thus "genera."

Noteworthy, try to be careful with plural words like data and media, which show a striking tendency to become wrongly singularized, probably because they look like singular feminine words. Remember they are plural forms and that their singular counterparts are datum and medium, respectively. In addition, some rare nouns like "species" and "series" do not change when pluralized.

Table 1: Some medical nouns and their plural forms

Singular	Plural	Meaning/examples
1) Latin nouns ending with -a are pluralized by making the noun end with -ae		
Alga	Algae	A group of photosynthetic organisms (e.g., seaweed)
Lamella	Lamellae	A plate-like structure in an animal
Larva	Larvae	Juvenile form many insects undergo before changing into adults
Maxilla	Maxillae	The bones forming the upper jaw
Pupa	Pupae	Is a life stage of some insects undergoing transformation after the larva stage and before the adult (imago) stage
Formula	Formulae	An entity constructed using symbols or a list of ingredients
Vertebra	Vertebrae	The bones that make up the backbone (the spine)
Tibia	Tibiae	Is the larger and longer of the two bones in the leg below the knee in humans and vertebrates (the other is the fibula)
Antenna	Antennae	Appendages used for sensing in arthropods
Latin nouns ending with -us are pluralized by making the noun end with -i		
Alumnus	Alumni	A graduate or former member of a school, college or university
Fungus	Fungi	A group of organisms that include yeasts and mushrooms
Tetanus	Tetani	A disease characterized by spasmodic contraction of muscles and death (spasmodic paralysis)
Nucleus	Nuclei	A central or essential part around which other parts are gathered
Radius	Radii	Straight line extending from the center of a circle to its edge
Stimulus	Stimuli	Something, such as a drug or an electrical impulse, that causes a response in an organism
Syllabus	Syllabi	The elements taught in a particular subject
Latin nouns ending with -um are pluralized by making the noun end with -a		
Curriculum	Curricula	The elements taught in a particular subject
Bacterium	Bacteria	Microorganisms that are invisible to the naked eye
Medium	Media	A thing through which something is carried or transmitted
Stratum	Strata	Any of several parallel layers or levels of something
Cilium	Cilia	Projecting threads on a cell, that beats rhythmically for movement of a fluid past the cell or movement of the cell through liquid
Datum	Data	Information
Flagellum	Flagella	A slender narrow outgrowth of the cells of many microorganisms that is used for locomotion
Operculum	Opercula	A plug of mucus that fills an opening
Ovum	Ova	The female reproductive cell (egg)

Singular	Plural	Meaning/examples
Table 1: Some medical nouns and their plural forms (*continued*)		
Sternum	Sterna	Breastbone
Tympanum	Tympana	The eardrum
Latin nouns ending with -is are pluralized by making the noun end with -es		
Basis	Bases	Foundation or something that acts as a support
Analysis	Analyses	The separation of something into its constituents in order to find what it contains, or examine individuals parts
Crisis	Crises	A situation or a period in which things are very uncertain, difficult and painful
Diagnosis	Diagnoses	The identification of an illness or disorder in a patient
Hypothesis	Hypotheses	A tentative explanation for a phenomenon, used as a basis for further investigation
Oasis	Oases	Fertile ground in a desert where the level of underground water rises to or near ground level
Paralysis	Paralyses	Loss of voluntary movement as a result of damage to nerve or muscle function
Parenthesis	Parentheses	The curved signs "( )"
Synthesis	Syntheses	The process of forming a complex compound through a series of one or more chemical reactions
Synopsis	Synopses	A condensed version of text, for example, a summary of the plot of a book or movie
Thesis	Theses	A proposition advanced as an argument or a subject for an essay
Axis	Axes	A imaginary straight line around which an object, such as the earth, rotates
Latin nouns ending with -on are pluralized by making the noun end with -a		
Phenomenon	Phenomena	A fact or occurrence that can be observed
Criterion	Criteria	An accepted standard used in making decisions or judgments about something
Ganglion	Ganglia	A structure that contains a dense cluster of nerve cell bodies
Protozoon	Protozoa	Free-living microscopic animals like the amoeba
Latin nouns ending with -x are pluralize by making the noun ends with -ces		
Appendix	Appendices	A blind-ended tube leading from the first part of the large intestine (cecum); or a collection of separate material at the end of a book
Index	Indices	An indicator or sign for something, like an alphabetic list of names, subjects, with references where they occur; typically found at the end of a book

Singular	Plural	Meaning/examples
Table 1: Some medical nouns and their plural forms (*continued*)		
Matrix	Matrices	An environment or material in which something develops; a surrounding media or structure
Thorax	Thoraces	The part of the body between the neck and the abdomen (cavity enclosed by the ribs)
Greek nouns ending with -ma are pluralize by adding -ta to their ends		
Stemma	Stemmata	A diagram like a family tree, showing relationships
Stigma	Stigmata	Shame or disgrace attached to something regarded as unacceptable
Stoma	Stomata	A tiny pore in the outer layer of a plant leaf that control the passing of water vapor and other gases
Exceptions to the rules described above		
Genus	Genera	A category in the taxonomic classification of organisms
Tooth	Teeth	Hard white bony objects arranged in two arched rows inside a human or vertebrate animal's mouth
Goose	Geese	A large waterfowl with long neck and webbed feet
Foot	Feet	The part of the leg below the ankle joint
Louse	Lice	A wingless insect that lives as a parasite on humans and other animals. They include blood-sucking lice
Mouse	Mice	A small rodent with long hairless tail found worldwide
Corpus	Corpora	The main body or mass of a structure
Child	Children	A young human being between birth and puberty
Man	Men	An adult male human being
Woman	Women	An adult human female
Nouns where the singular form is the same as the plural form		
Series	Series	A number of similar or related things coming one after another
Sheep	Sheep	A hoofed mammal with ribbed horns raised for wool and meat
Species	Species	A group of living organisms consisting of similar individuals capable of exchanging genes or interbreeding
Offspring	Offspring	The descendants of people, animals, or plants

PART 1:3 COMBINING STEMS, PREFIXES AND SUFFIXES

Here we will introduce the basic component of medical terms, which are stems, prefixes and suffixes. The stem (also called a root) of a medical term usually indicates an organ or a body part (see Table 2), which can be modified by a prefix or suffix, or both. Every medical term has a stem, just like everyday words. For example, in the words cooker and printer, "cook" and "print" are the stems; and the "-er" is the suffix in both words. Another example is the word terminology, which is made of the stem terminus and the suffix -logy. The stem terminus means word or expression, and the suffix -logy means the study of or the science dealing with. In most medical terms the same is seen. For example, in the medical terms hepatotoxic and neurotoxic, the stems hepato- and neuro- refer to the liver and nerve tissues, respectively. The suffix -toxic means a poisonous substance. Therefore, hepatotoxic and neurotoxic denote a toxin that damages the liver and the nervous system, respectively. Similarly, the suffix -cyte denotes cell. Thus, the term hepatocyte denotes a liver cell.

Certain combinations of stems, prefixes and suffixes could be hard to pronounce. This is true if the stem ends with a consonant and the word part that is added to it also begins with a consonant. A consonant is a speech sound produced by partly or totally blocking the path of air through the mouth. A consonant can be combined with a vowel to form a syllable. Thus, to remove the potential difficulty of pronunciation a combining vowel is simply inserted. The combining vowel between stems, prefixes and suffixes is most commonly an "o," but the vowels "i", "e", "u" or "y" are also occasionally used. We find combining vowels in ordinary words such as in the word "thermometer," which is made of the stem therm-, which means temperature, and the word meter, which means to measure. We insert the combining letter "o" to make it easier to pronounce the word "thermometer." In medical terminology, the suffixes and prefixes are primarily in Geek, but sometimes in Latin, and the "o" is almost always the combining vowel connecting the different parts of the medical term (see Figure 2). For example, arthrology is made of the stem arthr- which means joints, the combining "o" and the suffix -logy, which means science. Thus arthrology refers to the science dealing with joints. The stem plus a combining vowel are known as the "combining form." In the word thermometer the word therm is the stem and thermo is the combining form. Generally, the combining "o" is dropped when connecting to a vowel stem. For example, the medical term arthritis is made of the stem arthr and the suffix -itis, which means inflammation, without using the combining form arthro.

Basic Word Structure

1. Word root:

Gastr-

Root (stem) for ("stomach")

2. Suffix (word ending):

Gastritis   *Gastric*

Suffix ("inflammation")   Suffix ("pertaining to")

3. Prefix (word beginning):

Epigastric

Prefix ("above")

4. Combining vowel: a vowel usually "O" linking the root to suffix, prefix or another root:

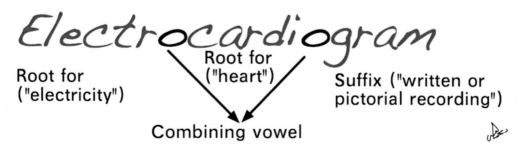

Electrocardiogram

Root for ("electricity")   Root for ("heart")   Suffix ("written or pictorial recording")

Combining vowel

Figure 2: Illustration of combining roots, prefixes and suffixes.

Table 2: Common roots for body parts

Body part	Medical stem
Abdomen	Lapro-
Aorta	Aort-
Arm	Brachi-
Armpit	Axill-
Artery	Arteri-
Back	Dors-
Bladder	Cyst-, vesic-
Blood	Haemat-, hemat-, haem-, hem-, -emia
Blood clot	Thromb-
Blood vessel	Angi-, vascul-, vas-
Body	Somat-, som-, corpor-
Bone	Oste-, ossi-
Bone marrow	Myel-, medull-
Brain	Encephal-, cerebr-
Breast	Mast-, mamm-
Chest	Steth-, thorax
Cheek	Bucc-
Ear	Ot-, aur(i)-
Egg, ova	Oo-, ov-
Eye	Ophthalm-, ocul-, optic-
Eyelid	Blephar-, cili-, palpebr-
Face	Faci-
Fallopian (uterine) tubes	Salping-
Fat, fatty tissue	Lip-, adip-
Forehead	Front-
Gallbladder	Cholecyst-
Genitals	Gon-, phall-
Gland	Aden-
Gums	Gingiv-
Heart	Cardi-
Intestine	Enter -
Joint	Arthr-
Kidney	Nephr, ren-, ur-
Lip	Cheil-, chil- labi-
Liver	Hepat-, -hepatic
public region	Episi-, pudend-
Lungs	Pneumon-, pulmo-, pulmon(i)-
Mind	Psych-
Mouth	Stomat-

Muscle	My-, sarco-
Navel	Omphal-, umbilic-
Neck	cervic-, trachel-
Nerve, nervous system	Neur-
Nose	Rhin-, nas-
Ovary	Oophor-,
Pelvis	Pyel-, pelv(i)-
Rib	Pleur-, cost-
Rib cage, chest cavity	Thorac(i)-, thorac-
Shoulder	Om-, humer-
Skin	Dermat-, derm-, cutaneous
Skull	Crani-
Stomach	Gastr-
Testis	Orchi-, orchid-
Tooth	Odont-, dent(i)-
Tongue	Gloss-, glott-, lingu(a)
Tumor	onc-, tum-, -oma
Urine, urinary system	Ur-, urin-
Uterus, womb	Hyster-, metr-, uter-
Vagina	Colp-, vagin-
Vein	Phleb-, ven-
Vulva	Episi-, vulv-

PART 1:4 TERMS FOR POSITION

The prefix intra- means inside or within. Recall from Table 2 that cerebro- means the brain, and intracerebral hemorrhage thus means bleeding inside the brain (Figure 3). This internal bleeding can lead to a stroke, which is a sudden disabling attack or loss of consciousness caused by an interruption in the flow of blood to the brain. Stroke is an increasingly common disease in modern societies such as Saudi Arabia. It usually leads to serious disability and death. Factors that can predispose to strokes include lack of physical activity (exercise) and high fat intake. Intracellular proteins refer to proteins inside the cell. Intravenous administration of a drug means the direct injection of a drug into a vein. Intraabdominal means inside the abdomen. The term endo- also means within or inside. And since metro- means uterus and -itis means inflammation, therefore endometritis means inflammation inside the uterus. Endoscopy means viewing the inside of the human body using an endoscope, an instrument made of optic fibers and equipped with a camera and a monitor. The term cardio- means heart, and therefore endocarditis means inflammation of the layers of tissues covering the inside the heart. The term -crine means to secrete. Therefore, an endocrine gland releases its secretions inside the body (into the blood stream). Also, the prefix en- means inside, and therefore encephalopathy is a disease in which the functioning of the brain is affected by some agent of condition, like a virus or toxin in the blood (cephalo- "head" + -pathy "disease").

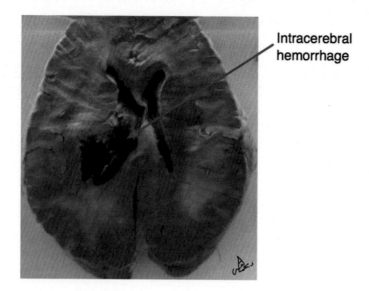

Intracerebral hemorrhage

Figure 3: A cross-section of a human brain containing an intracerebral hemorrhage.

On the other hand, ex(o)- means outside, and thus an exocrine gland release its secretions outside the blood (e.g., sweat glands). The prefix extra- also means outside; therefore, extracellular proteins are located outside the cells. Similarly, the extracellular matrix refers to the components that are located outside the cells to provide structural support in tissues. Ecto- also means outside. An ectopic pregnancy is a pregnancy that occurs outside the uterus. Abu Al-Qasim Al-Zahrawi (know in the west as Abulcasis) was the first physician to describe ectopic pregnancy.

Trans- is a prefix that means across, through or changes. Transcutaneous means to measure or apply something across the depth of the skin (cutaneous means skin). Transformation is a dramatic change in form or appearance. Transactivation is the activation of a gene at one locus by the presence of a particular gene on another locus, typically following infection by a virus. That is, the presence of the viral gene activates other genes across the genome. Transplantation means the move or transfer of something (e.g., an organ) to another place or situation.

Inter- as a prefix means between. Therefore, since the ribs are referred to with the stem costal, the intercostal muscles are the muscles located between the ribs. Similarly, the interventricular cardic artery is an artery that runs between the two ventricles of the heart. Dextr- means right sided. Dextrocardia is a congenital defect in which the heart is situated on the right side of the body rather than the left side. Levo- means left. Levoversion means the act of turning to the left. Retro- is a prefix that means behind. Therefore, a retrocardial infection means an infection located behind the heart. Peri- is a prefix that means around or surrounding. Pericarditis thus means inflammation of the layers surrounding the heart, because cardi- is the stem word for the heart and -itis is the suffix for inflammation. The term odont- means tooth, and thus periodontal tissues refer to the structures (ligaments and bones) surrounding and supporting the teeth, while periodontitis means inflammation of the ligaments and bones that support the teeth. Epi- is a prefix that means outermost or above. Thus, the epicardium is the outer layer covering the heart tissue and the epidermis is the outermost layer of the skin (the dermis is the thick layer of living tissue below the epidermis that forms the true skin, containing blood capillaries, nerve endings, sweat glands, hair follicles and other structures). The term gastric means stomach, and thus epigastric vessels are those located above the stomach. Sub- and hypo- mean under or below (low). Subcutaneous refers to a location below the skin (cutaneous is a term for the skin). Hypoglycemia is low blood glucose concentration. A hypodermic needle is one that is inserted below the skin's dermis. Hyper- is a prefix that means above or high. Hyperglycemia is an excess of glucose in the bloodstream, often associated with diabetes mellitus.

Terms used to describe location of body parts (Figure 4) include:

1. Superior: toward the head (above).
2. Inferior: away from the head (below).
3. Lateral: on the outer side (away from midline).
4. Medial: on the inner side (toward the midline).
5. Posterior: toward the back (behind).
6. Anterior: toward the front of the body.
7. Distal: away from the origin of a limb.
8. Proximal: toward the origin of a limb.

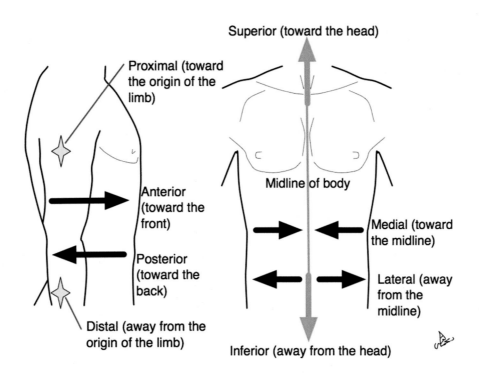

Figure 4: Illustration of the terms used to describe the location of body parts.

Therefore, since the term antero- means anterior (in front of), the anteroapical surface of the tongue is the anterior upper surface of the tongue. And since latero- means toward the side, anterolateral means located in front and toward the side. Similarly, since posterior means behind, an anteroposterior X-ray film views body parts from the front to the back. Mes- and medi- mean located in the middle. Mesaortitis means inflammation of the middle layer of the aorta, the largest blood artery in the human body. Mediastinum is the space in the chest between the plural sacs (where the lungs are enclosed). The mediastinum (Figure 5) contains all the viscera (organs) of the chest except the lungs and the pleurae (the sacs enclosing the lungs).

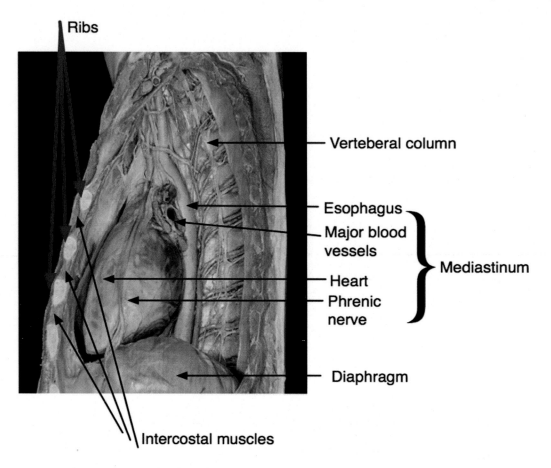

Figure 5: A sagittal-section of human thorax showing the mediastinum.

Studying body parts requires dissecting, and the directions of dissecting body planes have names that aid in understanding and communicating anatomical information. The body planes that are used to study the human body under dissection (Figure 6) include:

1. Median plane (midsagittal): separates the body into right and left parts.
2. Sagittal plane: any plane parallel to the median plane.
3. Horizontal (transverse) plane: separates the body into superior and inferior parts. Sometimes this plane is called a cross-section or an axial plane.
4. Frontal (coronal) plane: separates the body into anterior and posterior parts.

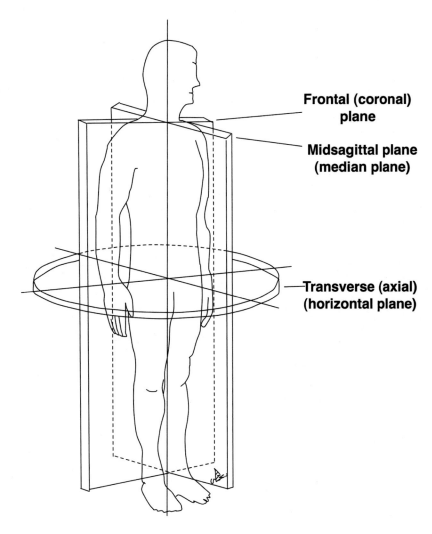

Frontal (coronal) plane

Midsagittal plane (median plane)

Transverse (axial) (horizontal plane)

Figure 6: Illustration of the terms used to describe the planes of the body.

Table 3: List of terms used for describing position

Description	Medical term
Around, surrounding	Peri-
Above, outer	Epi-, hyper-
Inside	Intra-, end-, em-, en-
Outside	Extra-, ecto-, ex-
Through, across, change	Trans-
Behind, before	Retro-, post-
Under, low	Sub-, hypo-, inferi-
Between	Inter-
Left	Levo-
Middle	Mes-, medi-
Right	Dextr-
In front	Anter-
In the side of	Later-
Behind	Posteri-

PART 1:5 TERMS FOR NEGATION

The prefixes a- and an- mean without, or the absence of. Accordingly since febrile means fever, afebrile means without fever. Also, since the stem aesthesia means sensation (feeling), thus anesthesia means without sensation. Similarly, since algesia means to feel pain, an analgestic drug is one that acts to relieve pain or stop the sensation of pain. Anemia is a condition marked by a deficiency of red blood cells or of hemoglobin (note that the prefix -emia means blood).

The prefixes in-, un-, im-, and il- similarly mean without. For example, involuntary means without volition (voluntary choice) and is especially used for muscles concerned in bodily processes that are not under the control of the will. For example, the muscles of the stomach are involuntary. Unconscious means without consciousness, that is, done or existing without realizing and feeling it (unaware of it). Because mobile means able to move, therefore, immobile means not moving or incapable of moving. Immobility can result from spinal cord injury. The word illegal means contrary to, or forbidden by law (criminal).

The prefix de- denotes removal or loss of. And since hydr- is the term for water, dehydrate is a verb meaning to lose a large amount of water. Since vital means life and activity, a devitalized tissue refers to dead tissue (tissue that has lost strength and life). Tooth decay (cavity) is due to bacterial acids, which cause the demineralization of the tooth surface. Demineralization means to remove minerals such as calcium and phosphorus, causing the tooth enamel to become soft and weak and thereby susceptible to decay (dental cavities). Demineralization can happen to any bone in the body. The disease known as osteoporosis (osteo- "bone" + por "porous or spongy" + -osis "condition") is a medical condition where the bones become weak, brittle, and fragile due to the demineralization of bone tissues, typically as a result of calcium or vitamin D deficiency.

The prefix pseudo- means false. Pseudomembrane is a layer of exudate resembling a membrane formed on the surface of the skin or of a mucous membrane. It gives the illusion a membrane is present, but in reality there is no actual membrane. Pseudoappendicitis is a condition characterized by symptoms and signs similar to those of appendicitis but not resulting from inflammation of the vermiform appendix.

The prefix ab- means not. Thus, abnormal means not normal or deviating from what is normal or usual, typically in a way that is undesirable or worrying. Likewise, the prefixes ir- and ar- mean not. For example, arrhythmia is a condition in which the heart beats with an abnormal rhythm. This condition is also commonly called irregular heartbeat. Similarly, an irreversible disease is one that is not reversible. Moreover, the prefix non- also means not. Thus, one can say water is a nontoxic, nonradioactive, and nonfatal substance. This means that water is not toxic, not radioactive, and not fatal. Other words that contain the prefix non-, include nonselective, noninvasive, and nonsustained. Some medications, like aspirin, are nonselective because they inhibit both inflammation and other body functions, such as the production of gastric mucus, possibly leading to stomach ulcers. Some bacteria are noninvasive because they remain localized. Nonsustained means short-lived.

The prefix dys- means bad, painful, incorrect, or not working. Dysphagia is the word for the symptom of difficulty of swallowing. Dysuria means difficult or painful urination. Mal- is a prefix meaning bad. Malodorous means having bad odor (smell). Oral malodor means bad mouth-breath. Malnutrition means lack of proper healthy food in the diet or excessive intake of unhealthy foods or being unable to use the food that one does eat, leading to physical harm (bad nutrition of the body). Malnutrition is common in both developed and developing countries. Malformation means an abnormally formed part of the body. Exposure to radiation during pregnancy can lead to malformations in the fetus.

The prefix mis- means incorrect, inaccurate, or wrong. Thus, a misdiagnosis is an incorrect diagnosis or assessment of a patient's condition. Harm may be caused as a result of an incorrect therapeutic intervention prescribed based on a misdiagnosis. Mismatch, in blood transfusion and transplantation medicine, means incompatibility between potential donor and recipient. That is; a state of not being able to exist in harmony and producing adverse effects because the donor and recipient blood groups conflict. Mismatch, in molecular biology, means that one or more nucleotides in the double-stranded, nucleic acid (e.g., DNA or RNA) are not complementary. Other words that contain the prefix mis- include mislabeled, misread, misunderstood, misplaced, and misused. Drugs can be very dangerous if they are mislabeled or misused. They are also a source of danger to children if they were misplaced. In addition, adults can harm themselves if they misread or misunderstand the labels on drugs.

Dis- means opposite of. Therefore, disability means a physical or mental condition that limits a person's abilities (movements, senses, or activities). Dislocation of a bone, means deviation from the proper or usual place, commonly occurring in injury when the normal position of a bone is put out of a joint (e.g., dislocation of the hip joint is common in the elderly). Similarly, disadvantage means an unfavorable circumstance or condition (the opposite of advantage). Moreover, disappear means cease to be visible (opposite of appear). Another example for the prefix dis- is discolor, which means to become a different, less attractive color, or to change or spoil the color. Disinfectant is a chemical liquid that destroys the causative agents of infection. These are bacteria, viruses, fungi, protozoa, and other parasites.

The prefix anti- means to act against, kill, or attack. Thus, an antitoxin (antidote) is something that acts against a toxin, and can thus be used to cure intoxication. An antitoxin is a type of antibody. An antibody is a protein produced by the immune cells to attack any foreign body (e.g., viruses, bacteria, or toxins). Antibiotics are drugs that kill bacteria, fungi, and other microorganisms (anti- "against" + biotic "living organism"). Antiarrhythmics are a group of medications used to stop (by acting against) cardiac arrhythmias.

Another prefix that means against is contra-. A contraceptive is a method, device, or drug serving to prevent pregnancy. That is, acting against pregnancy (the suffix -ceptive means conception, which refers to fertilization and pregnancy). Contraindication is any condition, which renders a particular line of treatment improper or undesirable. That is, any condition acting against the good outcomes desired from a treatment.

PART 1:6 TERMS FOR TIME

The prefixes pro-, ante-, and pre- mean before. A prophylactic measure refers to a medicine or course of action used to prevent disease before exposure to it. Antibiotics can be taken as prophylaxis against bacterial infections (pro "before" + phylaxis "act of guarding"). Thus prophylaxis means "an advance guard."

Antenatal means before childbirth, and preoperative medication is that which is administered before operation (surgery). Post- is a prefix meaning after or following. Thus, the term postoperative denotes after the surgical operation. A postoperative complication is a side effect of the operation that occurs after surgery. Postmenopausal means after menopause, which is the period of time after a woman has experienced no menstruations (typically after 45 or 50 years of age).

The prefix re- indicates a return to the previous condition, repetition of a previous action, or back to the original state again. Thus, a recurrent infection is any infection that occurs repeatedly. Also, reabsorption is the act of absorbing again, as in the absorption by the kidneys of substances (glucose, amino acids, salts) already secreted into the renal tubules. This is called reabsorption because these substances were already absorbed into the blood from the small intestine. The prefix co- means to happen together. Therefore, coexist means to exist at the same time and place. Coincubation means to incubate two things together. For example, some intracellular parasites, like viruses, must be coincubated with other cells to replicate. Noct- is a prefix meaning night. Nocturia means urination during the night, and nocturnally means done, occurring, or active at night (Table 4).

Table 4: List of terms used for describing (1) negation and (2) time.

Description	Medical term	Examples
(1) Terms describing negation		
Without or absence of	a-, an-, in-, un-, im-, il-	afebrile, anaesthesia, analgestic, anemia, insoluble, involuntary, unconscious, unlikely, unnatural, immobile, impossible, illegal
Removal of	de-	dehydrate, demineralization
False	pseudo-	Pseudomembrane
Not	ab-, ir-, ar-, non-	abnormal, irregular, arrhythmia, nontoxic, nonfatal, nonspecific
Bad, painful, or difficult	dys-, mal-	dysuria, dysphagia, malnutrition, malodor, malformation
Incorrect or wrong	mis-	misdiagnosis, mismatched
Opposite of	dis-	disability, dislocation, disappear
Against	anti-, contra	antibiotic, antitoxin, antibody, contraceptive, contraindication
(2) Terms describing time		
Before	pro-, ante-, pre-	prophylaxis, antenatal, preoperative
After or following	post-	postoperative
Again	re-	reabsorption, recurrent infection
Night	noct-	nocturia, nocturnal
Happen together	co-	coexist, coincubation

PART 1:7 TERMS FOR BODILY CONCEPTS

There are a few very common and important terms for bodily concepts (Table 5). One such important term is that for disease; -pathy or path-. Thus, pathology is the science dealing with diseases and the processes of a particular disease. For example, one can say: the pathology of cancer is hard to understand. Another example is seen in words like neuropathy, meaning pathology of neurons (nerve cells). Similarly, one can say encephalopathy, meaning pathology of the brain (en "inside" + cephalo "head"). Other examples include: myelopathy (pathology of bone marrow), lymphadenopathy (pathological enlargement of lymph nodes), and ophthalmopathy (pathology of the eye). Recall that the prefixes dys-, dis-, and mal- mean bad, painful, incorrect, or not working. Dysfunction means abnormality or impairment in the function of a specified bodily organ. Dystrophy is a disorder in which an organ or tissue of the body wastes away (note that the suffix -trophy means nourishment and growth). Disorient means to make someone lose their orientation (sense of direction), which is a common symptom in people that suffer from brain damage. Malabsorption means imperfect absorption of food material by the small intestine. Malabsorption can cause malnourishment, which means deficiency of the substances necessary for growth and health. The suffix for pain is -algia, which means to feel pain. Myalgia means pain in the muscle. Arthralgia means pain in the joints.

Another very important medical suffix is that used for inflammation; -itis. Dermatitis is inflammation of the dermis, which is the thick, sensitive layer of the skin beneath the epidermis. Meningitis (Figure 7) is an inflammation of the meninges, the layers covering the brain and the spinal cord (the meninges are three membranes (the dura mater, arachnoid, and pia mater) that line the skull and vertebral canal, enclosing the brain and spinal cord). Hepatitis is the inflammation of the liver (recall that hepat- denotes the liver). Pericarditis is an inflammation of the pericardium, the covering of the heart muscle (peri "surrounding something" + cardio "heart" + ium "tissue"). Carditis is inflammation of the heart itself. Myocarditis is inflammation of the heart muscle.

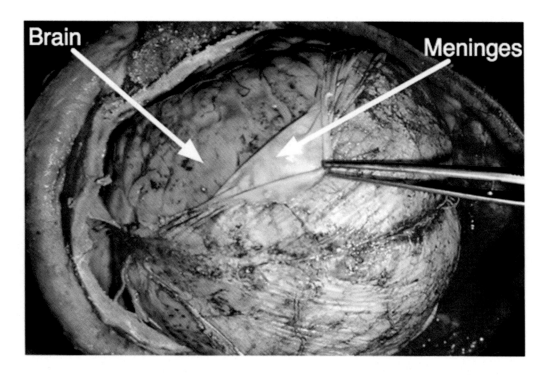

Figure 7: meningitis. Obtained from the Centers for Disease Control and Prevention.

Pyo- is the prefix for pus. Pyogenic bacteria are bacteria capable of causing pus to be formed. A pyocyst is a sac (cyst) containing pus. Pyomyositis means pus formation in muscles (suppurative myositis), pyoarthritis means inflammation and pus formation in joints, and a pyodermatous lesion is a skin lesion containing pus. Pyostomatitis (Figure 8) means pus formation on, and inflammation of, the mucus membranes of the mouth. Abscess is the name for a swollen area within the body containing accumulation of pus.

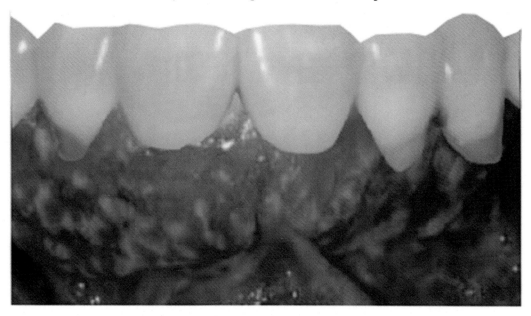

Figure 8: Pyostomatitis. Obtained from the Department of Microbiology and Immunology, University of Otago, Dunedin, New Zealand.

Necro- means dead. Spider venom can cause necrosis of human skin at the site of the bite and even systemic toxicity. Initial treatment includes cleansing, application of sterile dressing, cold compresses, and elevation and immobilization of the affected limb. In addition, the administration of dapsone, a leukocyte inhibitor, may stop the necrosis. Analgestics, anti-inflammatory drugs, and antibiotics can help prevent systemic complications. Febri- pertains to fever. Febrile flu refers to someone with flu symptoms and fever. Relapsing fever caused by the bacterium *Borrelia recurrentis*, and malaria caused by *plasmodium malariae*, can cause febrile intervals followed by afebrile intervals.

The prefix -plegia means paralysis. Thus, hemiplegia means paralysis (palsy) of half the body (hemi- means half). The term of involuntary contraction is -spasm. Therefore, myospasm, angiospasm, and bronchospasm mean involuntary contraction of muscles, blood vessels, and bronchi, respectively (myo- means muscle, angio- means blood vessel, and broncho- means bronchi, which are the major air passages of the lungs that diverge from the windpipe).

Suffixes such as -rrhea and -rrhage mean excessive flow of discharge. Thus, rhinorrhea is a condition known as runny nose (because rhin- means nose). It is characterized by a nasal cavity filled with mucous fluid. Similarly, hemorrhage is the discharge of blood from a ruptured blood vessel, especially when profuse (hem- means blood).

The suffixes -gen, -gensis, -poiesis, -trophy, and -plasia mean producing, formation, or growth. Thus, a pathogen is a bacterium, virus, or other microorganism that can produce disease. Similarly, angiogenesis is the development of new blood vessels (the prefix angio- means vessels). Erythropoiesis is the formation of red blood cells (erythro- refers to red blood cells). Hypertrophy is the enlargement of an organ or tissue (hyper- means over, high, beyond, above, or excessive). Atrophy means waste away, typically due to the degeneration of cells, or become smaller in size (recall that the prefix a- means without or absence of). Hyperplasia means excessive development or growth.

Neo- denotes new. Neoplasm means new and abnormal growth of tissue in some part of the body, especially as a characteristic of cancer (tumor). The suffix for cancer is -oma. And because adeno- means gland or glandular tissue, an adenoma is therefore a cancer formed from glandular tissue. The prefix for cancer is onco-. Oncology is the study of cancers and oncogenesis is the development of a cancer.

The suffix denoting a process or a condition is -osis. Thus, fibrosis is a process involving the thickening and scarring of tissue due to an increase in fiber content, usually as a result of injury. Thrombosis is a disease caused by the formation of thrombi (blood clots). Another suffix for condition, formation of, or presence of, is -asis. Since nephro- refers to the kidneys and -lithi- is the term for rocks, stones, or earth, nephrolithiasis is therefore the formation of stones in the kidneys.

The medical term for hardening is sclerosis. Thus, arteriosclerosis (also called atherosclerosis) is a disease characterized by the deposition of fatty material on the inner walls of arteries, causing them to thicken and harden. This is a common disease in modern society. The suffix -malacia means softening. Osteomalacia is a disorder characterized by defective bone mineralization, leading to weak and soft bones (note that oste(o)- means bone). The suffix -porosis means to become porous (having minute spaces or holes through which liquid or air may pass). Osteoporosis is a medical condition, in which the bones become brittle and fragile from loss of tissue, typically as a result of deficiency of calcium or vitamin D.

-Ectasis and -ectasia are suffixes meaning dilation or expansion. Angiectasis means abnormal dilation of a blood vessel. The suffix for prolapse or downward displacement is -ptosis. Since the term for eyelid is blepharo, blepharoptosis means downward displacement of the eyelid. The suffix -cele means hernia, protrusion, or tumor. A gasterocele then, is a protrusion or hernia of the stomach. The suffix for narrowing is -stenosis. Bronchostenosis refers to chronic narrowing of the bronchi, which are the major air passages of the lungs that diverge from the windpipe (the trachea).

Emesis means vomiting. Prevention of poison absorption can be achieved by administration of activated charcoal suspension in water, given orally. The charcoal absorb the ingested poisons within the gut lumen, allowing the charcoal-toxin complex to be sent away with stool. The complex can also be evacuated from the stomach by induced emesis. People with pathological emesis can be treated with antiemetic drugs. Hematemesis refers to vomit containing blood, which can occur in patients with esophageal or stomach cancer, or ulcer (recall that hemat- means blood). The suffix phage denotes eating. Thus, a macrophage is a phagocyte (phagocytic cell). That is, a cell that can eat and digest bacteria, viruses, foreign bodies, and cell debris.

Bardy- denotes slow and cardi- is the term for heart. Therefore, bardycardia means slow heart rate. Tachy- means fast. Thus, a person with tachycardia has an abnormally fast heartbeat. Micro- means small and -cyte is the suffix for cell, and a microcyte is thus a very small cell. A microorganism refers to microscopic (very small) organisms. Microcardia indicates small heart. Macro- is a prefix that means large. Macrocytes are large cells. Mega- also means large. A megacolon is an abnormally large colon. Pan- means total or all and hysterectomy means removal of the uterus. Thus, panhysterectomy is the complete removal of the uterus, i.e., complete hysterectomy. Since the suffix -demic means people, pandemic refers to something that is prevalent amongst all the people of a country or the world. A suffix for a deficiency or a decrease is -penia. And since leukocytes means white blood cells, thus leukocytopenia means a decrease in the numbers of white blood cells in the blood, leading to an increased risk of infection. Pancytopenia is a pronounced reduction in all the cells and formed elements of the blood (pan "all" + cyto "cell" + penia "deficiency").

The suffix -philia denotes fondness or love for a specific thing. Hydro- means water. Therefore, a hydrophilic substance is a one having a tendency to mix with, dissolve in, or be wetted by water. For example, salt and sugar are hydrophilic, since they dissolve in water easily. The opposite suffix is -phobic, which denotes extreme fear and aversion, or hatred and dislike. A hydrophobic substance is one that has a tendency to repel or fail to mix with water. Lipids and fats are hydrophobic substances. Molecules that have both a hydrophobic and hydrophilic moieties (parts), like phospholipids, are called amphipathic (Figure 9). The prefix amphi- means both. For instance, the word amphibian denotes a cold-blooded vertebrate animal of a class that includes frogs, toads, newts, and salamanders distinguished by having an aquatic, gill-breathing, larval stage followed by a terrestrial, lung-breathing, adult stage.

Lipo- and adipo- refer to fat or lipid. A lipoma is a tumor in fat tissue. Fat cells are called lipocytes or adipocytes (recall that the suffix -cyte denotes cell). Cholesterol is a lipid that your body needs to work properly, but too much cholesterol can increase your chances of getting heart disease. The medical term for high blood cholesterol is hyperlipidemia. Nonetheless, lipids are water insoluble, and are thus transported in blood as lipoproteins (lipids associated with proteins). Therefore, hyperlipoproteinemia is the more correct medical term for this disorder. Gluc- means glucose specifically and glyc- refers to any sugar that includes sugar polymers (carbohydrates). Glucocorticoids are a class of steroid hormones that play a role in regulating the metabolism of glucose (they also lower the immune reaction acting as anti-inflammatory). Glycosylation refers to the enzymatic addition of sugars. Glycolipids and glycoproteins are lipids and proteins to which sugars are attached, respectively.

Lipase is the name given to the enzyme that digests lipids. Note that the suffix -ase means enzyme. Thus, a nuclease is an enzyme that digests nucleic acids. A protease is an enzyme that digests proteins. The suffix for breakdown is -lysis. Hemolysis means the breakdown of red blood cells. Similarly, lipolysis, proteolysis, and glycolysis mean the breakdown of lipids, proteins, and glucose, respectively.

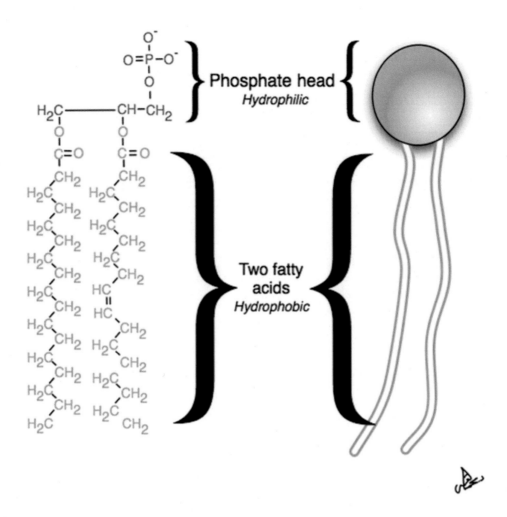

Figure 9: Illustration of the phospholipid amphipathic structure. Left; chemical structure, right; schematic representation.

The suffix for removing or excision is -ectomy. The term oophoro refers to the ovary. Thus, oophorectomy means the excision or surgical removal of one or both ovaries. Similarly, the term cholecyst means the gallbladder and cholecystectomy therefore means the surgical removal of the gallbladder. A term for fixation is -desis. Thus, arthrodesis means the surgical binding (repair) of a dislocated joint. Tenodesis is the surgical suturing of the end of a tendon to a bone. The suffix -pexy also mean fixation or suspension. Orchiopexy means fixation or suspension of an undescended testis (orchio- is the medical term for testis). Similarly, rectopexy means fixation of the rectum with a mesh or suture.

Table 5: Important terms describing bodily concepts

Description	Medical term
Bad, incorrect, disease	path-, pathy-, dis, dys-, mal-
Pain	-algia
Inflammation	-itis
Pus	Pyo-
Dead	Necro-
Fever	Febri-
Paralysis	-plegia
Involuntary contraction	Spasm
Discharge, excessive flow	-rrhea, -rrhage
Formation, production, or growth	-gen, -gensis, -poiesis, trophy, plasia
New	Neo-
Condition, process	-osis, -asis
Hardening	-sclerosis
Softening	Malacia-
Become porous	-porosis
Dilation or widening	-ectasis
Hernia or protrusion	-cele
Prolapse downward displacement	-ptosis
Narrowing	Stenosis
Vomiting	Emesis-, -emetic
Eating, ingesting or engulf	-phage
Slow	Brady-
Fast	Tachy-
Small	Micro-
Big, great	Macro-, mega-
Total, all	Pan-
Low, deficiency	-penia
Love, fondness	-philia
Hate, aversion	-phobia
Both	Amphi-
Fat	Lipo-, adipo-
Glucose, carbohydrates	Gluc-, glyc-
Water	Hydro-
Breakdown	-lysis
Excision	-ectomy
Fixation or suspension into place	-desis, -pexy

PART 1:8 TERMS FOR QUANTITY AND AMOUNT

Uni- and mono- are prefixes that mean one or single. Monotherapy for example refers to a treatment (therapy) that uses one drug. A monogenic inherited disease is one caused by one gene. A uninuclear cell is one that contains one nucleus. A unilateral headache refers to pain confined to one side of the head. A unicycle is a vehicle having one wheel.

Bis-, bi- and di- all mean two. Fructose 1, 6-bisphosphate is a fructose molecule phosphorylated on carbon 1 and 6, thus carrying two phosphate groups. Bilateral, therefore, means both sides. A bilateral mastectomy means surgical removal of both breasts (mast- means breast and -ectomy means excision). A bicycle is a vehicle having two wheels. Nicotinamide adenine dinucleotide (NAD), a vitamin known as niacin, contains two nucleotides. Similarly, riboflavin, vitamin B_2, is a flavin adenine dinucleotide. A phospholipid bilayer is a membrane made of two layers of phospholipids (Figure 11, page 31). In addition, diplo- means double. Diplopia means double vision, which is the simultaneous perception of two images for one single object. Cocci means spheres, and consequently, diplococci refers to two round cells attached together.

Tri- means three. A tricycle is a vehicle similar to a bicycle, but with three wheels. The valve of the heart, which has three folds (cusps), is called a tricuspid valve. A triacylglyceride is an ester derived from glycerol and three fatty acids and is the major constituent of animal fat and vegetable oil. Trisomy 21 (Down's syndrome) is a disease caused by the presence of three copies of chromosome 21 rather than the two normal copies. Tris- also means three. Inositol trisphosphate, an inositol to which three phosphates are attached, is a secondary messenger molecule used in single transduction within mammalian cells.

Quadri- and tetra- mean four. Quadriplegia means paralysis of the four limbs. The quadriceps muscle is a large muscle that is divided into four portions and is located in the front of the thigh. Tetra- also means four. Tetrahydrofolate (THF) is a folic acid derivative (a vitamin) that is hydrated at four locations.

Penta- means five. A pentanucleotide repeat is a repeat made of five nucleotides. Hexa- means six. Decohexanoic acid or docosahexaenoic acid is an omega-3 fatty acid with a chemical structure that includes six *cis* double bonds. It is found in fish and is important for brain functions. Omega-3 fatty acids are essential fatty acids that are very important for the development and wellbeing of the nervous system. Hepta- means seven. A heptapeptide is a peptide made from seven amino acids. Heptavalent antitoxin is an antitoxin active against seven versions of a toxin. Octo- means eight. The octopus is an animal with eight limbs.

Multi- and poly- mean many or much. Polynuritis means inflammation of many nerves. A disease that is caused by the combination of many factors is called a multifactorial disease.

A multinucleated cell is one that contains many nuclei (Figure 10). A polymer is a substance that has a molecular structure consisting of a large number of similar units bonded together like plastics (-mer means shared or similar). A polysaccharide is a molecule made of many saccharides units attached together. Polygeneic disorder is one caused by many genes that act together to create the disorder. On the other hand, oligo- is the prefix for little or few. Oligosaccharide is a molecule made of few saccharides. Oligoarthritis means inflammation of few joints.

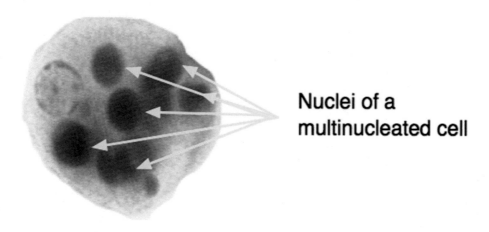

Nuclei of a
multinucleated cell

Figure 10: A multinucleated cell.

Tachy- means fast or many. A person with tachycardia has an abnormally fast heartbeat. Brady- refers to slow or few. A person with abnormally low heartbeat is said to have bradycardia. A suffix for deficiency or a decrease is -penia. Since thrombocytes means platelets, thrombocytopenia means a decrease in the numbers of platelets in the blood leading to bleeding into the tissues, bruising and slow blood clotting after injury. Also, hypo- means low. Therefore, hypothermia is a condition of having an abnormally low body temperature. Hyper- means high. Thus, hyperthermia is a condition of having body temperature greatly above normal. Recall that the term therm means temperature, and -ia means pertaining to.

Semi- and hemi- mean half. Hemiplegia means paralysis on one side of the body. The left brain hemisphere means the left half of the brain. Someone who is semiconscious is only half conscious. Semi- also means similar to. For example, semidesert area is a place that resembles a desert. A semiclosed building is an area with little ventilation. The prefixes equi- and iso- mean equal to. Equiangular means having equal angles. Isoenzyme is one enzyme in a group of two or more enzymes with identical functions but found in a different location and with a slightly different structure.

Table 6: Terms used to describe quantity and amount

Description	Medical term
Double	Diplo-, dupli-
Equal	Iso-, equi-
Few	Oligo-
Half	Hemi-, semi-
Many	Poly-, multi-
Fast	Tachy-
Slow	Brady-
Deficiency, decrease, lower	-penia, hypo-
Increase, beyond, exceeding	Hyper-
One	Uni-, mono-
Two	Bis, bi-, di-, dis-, dy-
Three	Tri-, tris-
Four	Tetra-, quadri-, quadru-
Five	Penta-
Six	Hexa-
Seven	Hepta-, septm-, septi-
Eight	Octo-, octa-
Nine	Novem-, ennea-, nona-
Ten	Decem-, dec-, deca–

PART 1:9 TERMS FOR COLOR

The prefix for color is chromo-. Thus, photochromogenic bacteria are a type of bacteria that can produce color when exposed to light (photo- "light" + -genic "producing"). Chromosomes are macromolecules that appear pigmented (colored) under the microscope and carry the genetic information in humans and other organisms.

The prefix leuko- and alb- mean white. Leukocytes are white blood cells. Albinism is a congenital disorder (inherited disease) characterized by the complete absence of pigment in the skin, hair and eyes. An organism with this condition is called an albino. Erythro- is a prefix meaning red. An erythrocyte, thus, refers to a red blood cell. Rhod- is another term for red. Rhodopsin is the name given to a red pigment in the retina of the eye that can absorb light and activates the vision receptors. Rubro- also means red. The rubrospinal tract is a band of nervous tissue connecting the red nucleus in the midbrain to the spinal cord. Cyano- is a prefix meaning blue. Cyanosis is the appearance of a blue discoloration of the skin and mucous membranes due to a lack of oxygenation. Cyanobacteria are blue-green bacteria that commonly grow in sunny aquatic environments. Melano- means dark or black. Melanoma is a malignant tumor comprised of melanocytes, which are cells that produce the dark pigment melanin that is responsible for the color of skin. Nigr- is another prefix meaning black. The substantia nigra (which means the black substance), is a structure located in the midbrain that plays an important role in reward, addiction and movement in human beings.

Chloro- means green. Chloroplasts are green organelles found in plant and algae cells that carry photosynthesis, which is the production of sugar from carbon dioxide and water though the use of sunlight as a source of energy. Chloroplasts are responsible for the green color of plants and algae. Xantho- means yellow. Xanthoma is a condition in which yellowish cholesterol-rich material is deposited in the tendons, skin and other body parts. Flav- is another prefix that means yellow. The group of flaviviruses is named after one member that causes yellow fever. The yellow fever in turn was named because of its propensity to cause yellow jaundice in its patients. Cirrho- denotes red-yellow in color. Cirrhosis is a chronic liver disease characterized by fibrosis, scar tissue formation and regenerative nodules making the liver often appear yellowish-red (orange) in color.

Table 7: Terms used to describe color

Color	Medical term	Example
Color	Chromo-	Chromosomes
Black	Melano-, nigr-	Melanoma
Blue	Cyano-	Cyanosis
Green	Chlor-	Chloroplasts
Red	Erythr-, rhod-, rub-, rubr-	Erythrocyte, Rhodopsin, rubrospinal tract
Red-yellow (orange)	Cirrh-	Cirrhosis
White	Leuc-, leuk-, alb-	Leukocytes, Albinism
Yellow	Xanth-, flav-	Xanthoma, flaviviruses

PART 1:10 TERMS FOR BODY STRUCTURE

Living beings are made of, from simplest to most sophisticated, atoms (like C, N, O, H and P), that make molecules (like amino acids, sugars, fatty acids), that make up macromolecules (like proteins, cellulose, and phospholipids), that make up organelles (like the cell membrane, mitochondria, lysosomes and golgi body), that make up cells, that make up tissues (connective tissue, epithelium and muscular), that make up organs (liver, heart and kidneys), that make up body systems (like the digestive system, respiratory system and the cardiovascular system), that make up the whole organism. A central theory in biology is cell theory, which is the outcome of many scientific experiments. Cell theory states:

(1)   All organisms are made of one or more cells.

(2)   Cells are the structural and functional unit of all organisms.

(3)   All cells come from a preexistent cell.

Cyto- is the prefix for cell. Cytology is the science that studies cells and their organelles. Organelle (-elle means small) denotes any structure within a living cell. -lemma is the suffix for membrane. The cell membrane, an organelle that surrounds the cell plasma, is called the plasmalemma. The plasmalemma and all other cellular membranes are made of molecules that join together making macromolecules. These include phospholipids, glycolipids, glycoproteins, proteins and cholesterol. The major macromolecule that makes the plasmalemma is phospholipid. The phospholipids are arranged as a bilayer (remember that bi- means two, and membranes are thus made of two layers of phospholipids). Phospholipids can form the lipid bilayer because there are amphipathic. That is, they contain a hydrophilic moiety (the phosphate group) and a hydrophobic moiety (the fatty acid tails). Figure 9 in page 25 depicts the structure of phospholipid. The phosphate groups face the water outside or inside the cell while the fatty acid tails point toward the center of the lipid bilayer. Figure 11 shows the lipid bilayer structure of the plasmalemma.

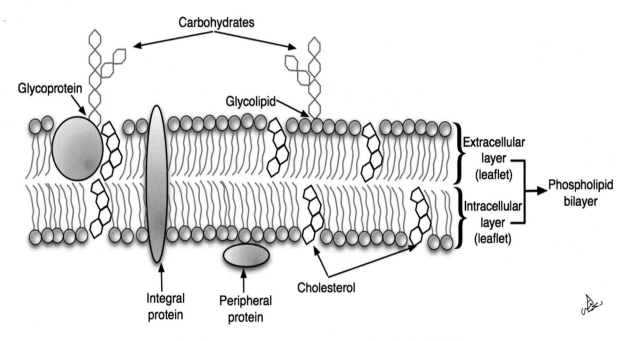

Figure 11: Illustration of the cell membrane phospholipid bilayer structure.

In addition, the cell organelles include the nucleus, which contains the nucleolus and the chromosomes (chromo "color" + some "body"). The nucleolus is where RNA is synthesized. RNA (ribonucleic acid) is an important macromolecule used for the synthesis of proteins. The chromosomes are made of DNA (deoxyribonucleic acid), which contains the code needed for the synthesis of RNA (ribonucleic acid) and, consequently, proteins. This is called the central dogma of biology describes this flow of information in biological systems. That is, DNA directs the synthesis of RNA in the nucleus through a process called transcription. Then, RNA directs the synthesis of proteins through the process called translation.

Karyo- denotes the nucleus of the cell. Karyotype refers to the number and visual appearance of the chromosomes in the cell's nuclei of an organism or species. Another cell organelle is the lysosome, which is a membrane bounded organelle containing hydrolytic enzymes for digestion of materials (lyso- "digestion" + -some "body"). The cell also contains the endoplasmic reticulum, which is a network of membranous tubules within the cytoplasm (endo- "within" + -plasmic "plasma" + reticulum "plural form of reticule which means "small tube or network" e.g., network of tubules"). The endoplasmic reticulum can be smooth (contains no ribosomes) or rough (contains ribosomes). Ribosomes are organelles responsible for protein synthesis and contain ribonucleic acid, hence their name (ribo- "ribonucleic acid" + -some "body"). Mitochondrion (plural: mitochondria) is the organelle where respiration and energy production occurs.

The golgi body is an organelle that modifies proteins received via transitional vesicles from the endoplasmic reticulum and secretes them outside the cell through secretory vesicles. The proteins can be modified by the addition of lipids or carbohydrates. That is, the golgi body can modify proteins to lipoproteins and glycoproteins. Peroxisomes are detoxifying organelles (note that de- means to remove and thus a detoxyifing organelle is one which removes toxins). Peroxisomes contain the enzyme catalase that breaks down the toxic hydrogen peroxide into water and oxygen (peroxi "hydrogen peroxide" + some "body"). Figure 12 shows some of the most important organelles inside the mammalian cell.

There are many types of cells in the human body. The suffix for cell is -cyte. Recall that adipo- and lipo- are prefixes for lipid or fat. Thus, adipocytes or lipocytes are cells specialized in storing fat. -blast is the suffix used to describe building cells that produce the extracellular matrix. For example, the medical suffix for bone is osteo-, and thus cells that build up bone extracellular matrix are called osteoblasts. Similarly, fibroblast denotes a cell that makes fibers such as collagen, which is a major component of tendons and ligaments. The suffix -clasts means breaking down; thus osteoclasts are cells that break down bone tissue. The suffix -phage means eating or engulfing, and macrophages are hence large immune cells (recall that macro- means large) that can engulf and eat bacteria, viruses, foreign bodies and cell debris.

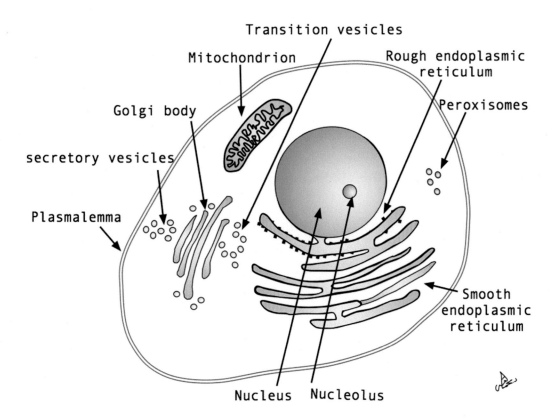

Figure 12: Illustration of the mammalian cell structure and organelles.

Cells come together and form tissues. There are four main types of tissues. These are the epithelium, connective, muscular and nervous tissues. The nervous tissue is made of two types of cells: neurons and neuroglia (neuro- "nerve" + glia "glue"). The neurons are the excitable nerve cells while the neuroglia are supportive cells that hold the neurons in position, protect them and provide them with nourishment. Neuroglia include the Schwann cells that form myelin sheaths around the axons of neurons (Figure 13).

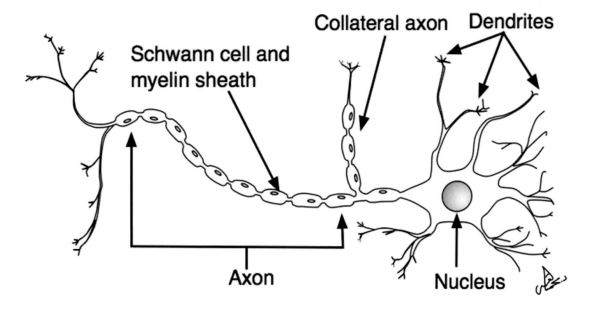

Figure 13: Illustration of the nerve cell, the neuron.

Epithelium (plural: epithelia) is made of close-packed cells covering body surfaces and lining cavities and forming glandular structures. There are two major types of epithelia: (1) epithelia covering and lining organs and (2) glandular epithelia that make up the secretary glands. The name of any given epithelium is derived from its structure (Figure 14) and includes the following.

(1) Simple: signifies an epithelium made of one layer.

(2) Stratified: signifies that the epithelium is made of multiple layers of cells (e.g., skin epidermis).

(3) Pseudostratified: signifies that the epithelium is made of one layer but appears as if there are multiple layers of cells (e.g., respiratory epithelium) because some cells reach the tissue surface while others do not, thus making their nuclei become visible in multiple layers given the illusion of stratification.

(4) Squamous: signifies flat (plate-like) cells.

(5) Columnar: signifies elongated cells (column shaped cells).

(6) Cuboidal: signifies cubical cells.

(7) Transitional: signifies that the cells can stretch many times their original size (e.g., the epithelium lining the urinary bladder).

(8) Keratinized: signifies the presence of dead cells on the outermost layer of the epithelium for the protection of the cells in the lower layers, as seen in human skin. The epithelium of the human skin is therefore called stratified squamous keratinized epithelium.

Mucous membranes (or mucosae; singular mucosa) are linings made of non-keratinized epithelium, which are involved in absorption, secretion and protection of body organs. They line cavities and areas that are exposed to the external environment and internal organs. They are located in several places neighboring the skin, such as in the nostrils, the mouth and lips, eyelids (conjunctiva), genital areas and anus. In addition, they line the gastrointestinal, the respiratory and the urinary tracts. The mucous membranes and its glands usually secrete a thick, sticky fluid called mucus. Mucus helps lubricate, moisten and protect mucous membranes. This is especially important for the gastrointestinal tract (from the mouth to the anus) and the respiratory tract (from the nose to the lungs). Another medical term commonly used for mucus is myxa. Thus, orthomyxoviridae (ortho "straight" + myxa "mucus" + viridae "viruses") are a family of viruses that include the human influenza virus, which is capable of attacking mucous membranes. Similarly, paramyxoviridae (para "beyond" + myxa "mucus" + viridae "viruses") are a family of viruses that include the human parainfluenza virus, measles and mumps. All these viruses can target mucus producing glands and membranes.

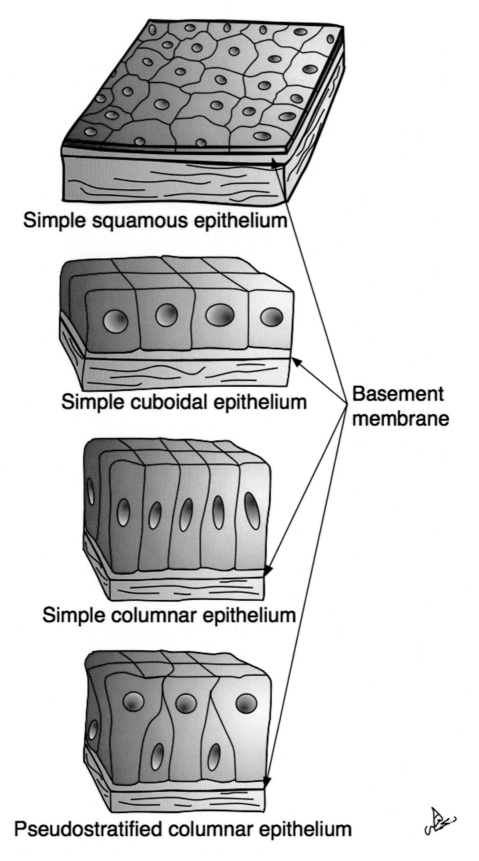

Simple squamous epithelium

Simple cuboidal epithelium

Basement membrane

Simple columnar epithelium

Pseudostratified columnar epithelium

Figure 14: Types of simple epithelia.

Connective tissue links, separates, supports and protects the body parts and organs. There are different types of connective tissue with varying degrees of fluidity, elasticity or rigidity. Examples include blood, bone, cartilage, tendons and ligaments. All connective tissues contain cells, which manufacture a matrix of extracelluar components including collagen, elastic fibers and amorphous glycosaminoglycans. Fibroblasts are commonly found in connective tissues.

Muscle tissue is made of cellular fibers capable of contracting to cause bodily movements. They are divided into skeletal, smooth and cardiac muscular tissues (Figure 15). Skeletal muscles are made of long, cylindrical, unbranched cells, called myofibers. Myofibers are arranged parallel in longitudinal tissue sections and contain striations. Each myofiber contains multiple nuclei near the periphery of the cells, immediately under the plasma membrane. The second type of muscle tissue is cardiac muscle. Cardiac muscle is only found in the heart and makes up its muscular tissue. The cells of this are short brunched cells (myocytes) that are less parallel than skeletal muscles and contain striations, intercalated discs and one centrally located nucleus per cell. The intercalated discs are the two membranes (plasmalemma) of the two adjacent myocytes attached together and containing gap junctions allowing for synchronized contraction of the entire heart muscle. Gap junctions are attachment sites between the membranes that form passage gates for ions and molecules to pass from one cell to the other. These passage gates are therefore communication channels for the cells to act as one unit. The third type of muscle tissue is called smooth muscles. These are short fusiform cells overlapping each other, non-striated, and each contains one centrally located nucleus. They usually form sheets of tissues in walls of viscera like the gastrointestinal, respiratory and urinary systems and in the walls of vessels (arteries and veins). The cardiac and smooth muscles are involuntary muscles. That is, they are not controlled consciously, whereas the skeletal muscles are voluntary muscles that are controlled consciously. The smooth and cardiac muscles usually contain nerves and nerve-like structure within them, whereas the only nerve supply to the skeletal muscles comes from the central nervous system (the brain and spinal cord). Therefore, injury to the spinal cord can lead to paralysis of the skeletal muscles but the cardiac and smooth muscles can remain active.

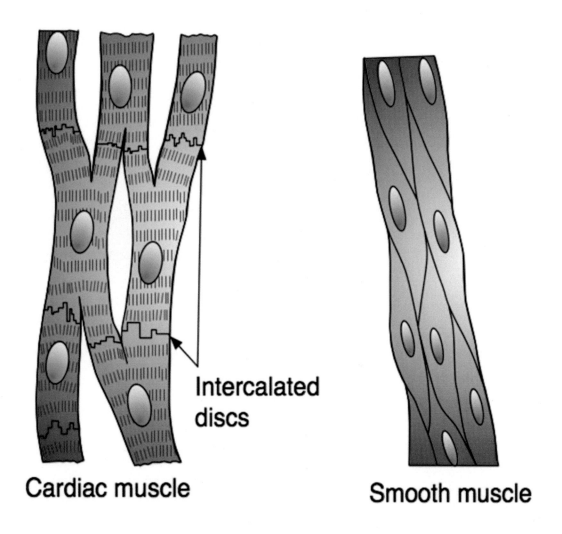

Intercalated discs

Cardiac muscle

Smooth muscle

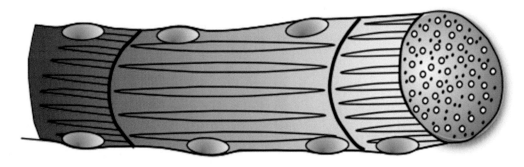

Muscle fiber or myofiber (single multinucleated skeletal muscle cell)

Figure 15: Types of muscle tissues.

PART 1:11 REVIEW QUESTIONS

As a review, write the meaning for each of the following:

1. intra/endo: _____
2. peri: _____
3. ec/ecto: _____
4. em/en: _____
5. retro/post: _____
6. antero: _____
7. sub/hypo: _____
8. a-: _____
9. anti-: _____
10. an-: _____
11. ante: _____
12. post-: _____
13. pre-: _____
14. ante-: _____
15. inter-: _____
16. pyo-: _____
17. lipo-: _____
18. febri-: _____
19. -itis: _____
20. necro-: _____
21. -emesis: _____
22. gluco-: _____
23. glycos-: _____

To exercise what you have learned, fill the blanks with the appropriate words:

1. Intrabdominal means _____.
2. Inflammation of the uterus is called _____.
3. Pericarditis is inflammation of _____.
4. The location behind the heart is called _____.
5. A needle inserted below the skin is called _____.
6. Antenatal means _____.
7. A preoperative medication is one given _____ surgery while a postoperative medication is one given _____ surgery.
8. The muscles located between the ribs are called _____.
9. Postnasal means _____ the nose.

10. Afebrile means without _____.

11. Loss of sensation due to preoperative medication is called _____.

12. Antitoxin is a medication used to cure _____.

13. Macrocytes are very _____ while microcytes are very _____.

14. Megacolon means _____.

15. Anterolateral means _____ while anteromedial means_____.

16. Pyogenic bacteria cause _____.

17. Cancer originating from lipocytes is called _____.

18. Someone without fever can be described as _____.

19. Necrosis is _____.

20. Hematemesis refers to the vomiting of _____.

21. Muscles tissues are divided into _____, _____ and _____ muscular tissues.

22. Glycosylation is the addition of _____ to _____.

To exercise what you have learned, describe the differences between the following prefixes or suffixes:

1. Intra- and inter-:_____

2. Hyper- and hypo-:_____

3. Extra- and intra-:_____

4. Micro- and macro-:_____

5. Post- and pre-:_____

6. Epi- and peri:- _____

7. Tachy- and brady-:_____

8. -phobic and -philic: _____

CHAPTER 2

THE MUSCULOSKELETAL SYSTEM

Chapter Contents

PART 2:1 INTRODUCTION

The musculoskeletal system, also known as the locomotor system, allows the body to move (locomote) using muscular, skeletal and fibrous components. In addition, the musculoskeletal system provides shape, support, protection, stability and locomotion (movement) for the body. The skeletal part of the system serves as the main storage site for calcium, phosphorus and other minerals. It is also the home for the hematopoietic tissue (hemato "blood" + poietic "forming"), the tissue responsible for making blood cells and blood components (e.g., red blood cells, white blood cells and platelets). The hematopoietic tissue is found in the bone marrow.

The musculoskeletal system is made of bones (that make up the skeleton), muscles, cartilages, tendons, and ligaments (Figure 16). The muscles are made of contractile cells. The bones are made of living cells embedded in a mineralized matrix of calcium phosphate and collagen fibers. Muscles are attached to bones via tendons. Ligaments attach bones to each other. Tendons and ligaments are two types of fibrous tissue, which contains fibrocytes, fibroblasts and collagen fibers. Joints, the meeting points between bones, are commonly called articulations. Articulations can be fixed or mobile. Fixed articulations allow no movements and include the sutures of the skull and the joints holding the teeth in position (Figure 18). Cartilages are commonly found between the bones in mobile joints. They act as cushions between the bones, absorbing shocks, and allowing for lubrication. The human skeleton contains 206 bones and is divided into two parts: the axial and appendicular skeletons.

In forensic medicine, the condition of the victim's bones can be used to derive valuable evidence about the committed crime, time of death and the age and sex of the victim. One of the common diseases that affect the skeletal system is osteoporosis. It is defined as a reduced mineralization (low calcium phosphate content) in the bones, causing them to become porous and weak. Osteoporosis is usually caused due to dietary insufficiencies of calcium, phosphate, vitamin D or vitamin C. The end result is weak bones that are highly susceptible to fractures. A balanced nutritious diet is therefore very important for healthy bones. In addition, exposure to sun rays allows the skin to synthesize vitamin D. More details about osteoporosis are outlined below.

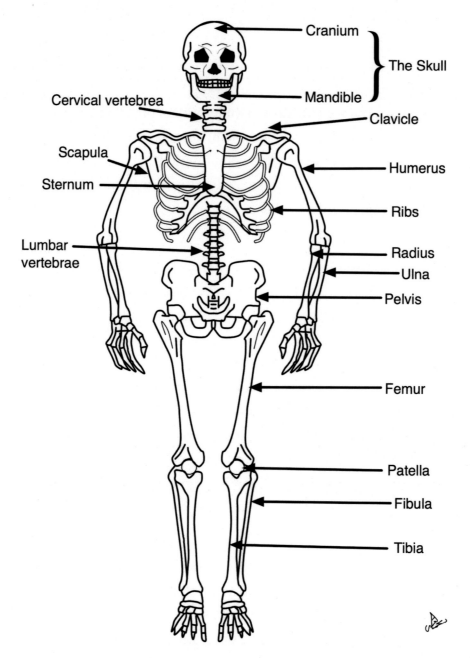

Figure 16: Illustration of the human skeleton.

PART 2:2 TERMS SPECIFIC TO THE MUSCULOSKELETAL SYSTEM

The skeleton is divided into axial and appendicular skeletons. The axial skeleton consists of the skull, the vertebral column, the sternum and the ribs. The appendicular skeleton consists of the bones of the lower and upper limbs and the girdles. The girdles are the bones of the shoulders (pectoral girdle) and the hips (pelvic girdle).

Osteo- is the medical term for bones. The term arthr- means joints. Thus, a person suffering from osteoarthritis has an inflammation of his bones and joints. The term chondro-means cartilage. Thus, chondritis means inflammation of cartilage. The term myo- means muscle. For example, myospasm means involuntary contraction of a muscle (spasm means involuntary contraction) and myopathy refers to disease (pathology) in muscles (recall that -pathy means disease). The term myelo- means bone marrow. Thus, myelitis means inflammation of bone marrow. Osteomyelitis means inflammation of bone and bone marrow. Remember that arthr- is the stem for joint. The term -desis means fixation. Thus, arthrodesis means fixation of a joint. It is a surgical procedure performed on two bones to fix a joint, such as an ankle, elbow or knee. This surgical procedure is used to treat severe arthritis or a damaged joint. Tenodesis is the surgical suturing of the end of a tendon to a bone. Tendonitis means inflammation of a tendon.

Recall that chondro- pertains to cartilages and costo- pertains to ribs. Therefore, a costochondral joint is a joint between a rib and a cartilage. The term thoracic describes the rib cage and the chest. And since intra- is a prefix for inside, intrathoracic pressure refers to pressure inside the rib cage.

Table 8: List of common terms used for describing musculoskeletal components

Root	Refers to	Example
Arthr-	Joint	Arthritis: inflammation of a joint
Myel-	Bone marrow	myelitis: inflammation of bone marrow
Chondr-	Cartilage	Chondritis: inflammation of cartilage
Cost-	Rib	costochondral joints: joints between a rib and a rib cage cartilage in the thorax
Crani-	Cranium/skull	intracranial: inside the skull
Oste-	Bone	Osteomyelitis: inflammation of the bone and bone marrow
Myo-	Muscle	Myospasm: involuntary contraction of muscles
Tend- or Teno-	Tendon	Tendonitis: inflammation of tendon

PART 2:3 THE BONES

Bone or skeletal medical specialists include orthopedic surgeons, osteopaths and rheumatologists. Osteology is the study of bones. Orthopedics is the branch of medicine dealing with the correction of deformities of bones or muscles. Osteopathy is a branch of medical practice that emphasizes the treatment of medical disorders through the manipulation and massage of the bones, joints and muscles. A rheumatologist is a medical specialist who deals with osteoarthritis, and other disorders of the joints, muscles and ligaments.

Osteogenesis means bone formation. Another name of bone formation is ossification. Calcification is the name given to the process of mineralization of the bone matrix (hardening). Bone tissue is made of an extracellular matrix and cells. The bone cells include osteocytes, osteoclasts and osteoblasts. Osteoclasts are cells that break down bone tissue (-clast means to break) and osteoblasts are cells that build bone tissue (-blast means to build). Osteoblasts secrete collagen fibers and other matrix components, which then harden by calcification, trapping the cells, which are then called osteocytes. Osteocytes are therefore trapped in cavities within the calcified matrix, known as lacunae. Osteocytes maintain the calcified matrix and receive nutrients from blood vessels via very small channels through the matrix called canaliculi. Osteoclasts are important in bone remodeling and renewal. They can break down calcified bone matrix and thus allow for the renewal and remodeling of bone tissue.

A common bone disease is osteoporosis (recall that osteo- means bone), and porosis means to become porous. Therefore, osteoporosis is a disease causing bones to become light, weak, porous and thinner because of an increase in the activity of osteoclasts compared to osteroblasts. Usually there is a balance between the two to allow for bone tissue renewal and strength. Osteoporosis (due to the weakness of bones) causes an increase in fractures (mainly in weight-bearing bones like the femur and the vertebrae) and therefore disabilities (morbidity). The disease is associated with ageing, poor calcium or vitamin D intake, lack of exercise, and smoking. It is more common in postmenopausal women in whom blood estrogen is low. It is medically recommended to have a good diet (containing enough calcium, phosphorus, vitamins and proteins), receive enough sun (for vitamin D synthesis by the skin) and to perform regular physical activities (to stimulate osteoblasts activity) to achieve peak bone mass in early life and prevent osteoporosis when elderly. In Saudi Arabia, more than 60% of the population suffers from vitamin D deficiency. Women are more susceptible because cultural constrains restrict their exposure to sun and their physical activity. Thus, it is recommended to take vitamin D supplements in regular basis. Some dairy products in Saudi Arabia are already fortified with vitamin D. In addition, fish and nuts are good sources of natural vitamin.

Long bones are made of a head, neck and shaft (Figure 17). Every bump, groove or hole on your bones has a name. There are two major categories of bone markings: projections (processes) and depressions, but each category includes many types (Table 9).

Table 9: List of terms used for describing bone markings

Type	Term	Definition
Projection	Condyle	Refers to a rounded articular projection
	Head	Is a bony projection on a narrow neck
	Facet	Smooth, nearly flat articular surface
	Ramus	Is an armlike bar of bone
	Epicondyle	Raised area on or above a condyle
	Tubercle	Small rounded projection
	Tuberosity	Large roughened projection or area
	Trochanter	Very large projection (only in femur)
	Spine	Sharp pointed projection
	Protuberance	Prominent projection
Depression	Meatus	Canal, tube or opening
	Fossa	Shallow basin
	Fissure	Narrow slit-like opening
	Sinus	Cavity within a bone, filled with air and lined with mucus membrane
	Foramen	Rounded or oval opening

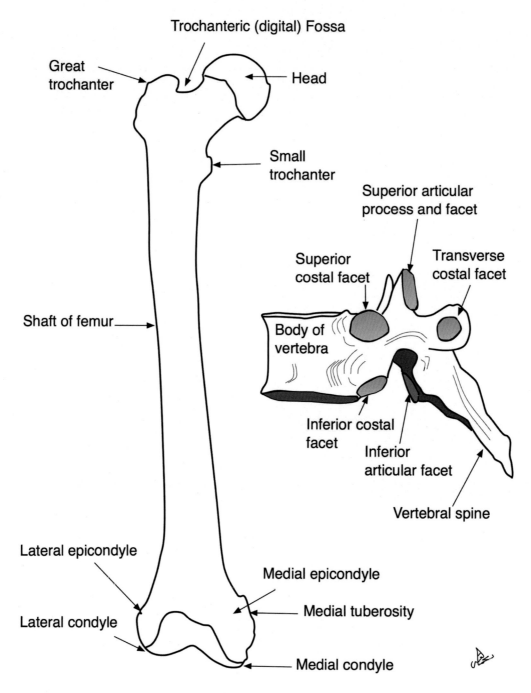

Figure 17: Illustration of the femur and a thoracic vertebra depicting their markings.

The skull is made of the cranium and the mandible. The cranium encloses the brain. The mandible is a horseshoe-shaped bone that forms the lower jaw. The cranium is made of several bones that are connected by immobile joints called sutures. These bones include the sphenoid, maxilla, frontal, parietal, temporal, occipital, zygomatic, lacrimal and nasal bones.

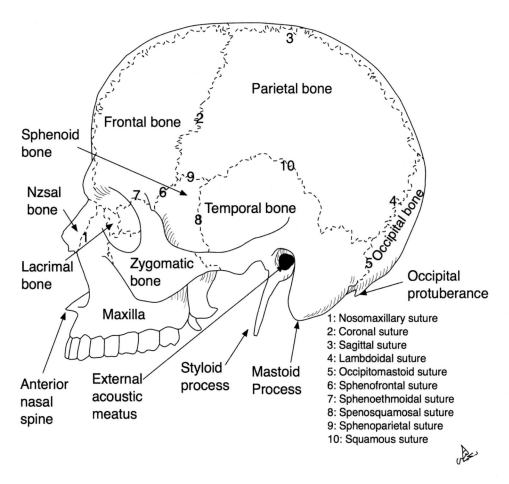

Frontal bone
Sphenoid bone
Parietal bone
3
2
10
9
6
7
Temporal bone
8
Nzsal bone
Occipital bone
5
4
Lacrimal bone
Zygomatic bone
Occipital protuberance
Maxilla
Styloid process
Mastoid Process
Anterior nasal spine
External acoustic meatus

1: Nosomaxillary suture
2: Coronal suture
3: Sagittal suture
4: Lambdoidal suture
5: Occipitomastoid suture
6: Sphenofrontal suture
7: Sphenoethmoidal suture
8: Spenosquamosal suture
9: Sphenoparietal suture
10: Squamous suture

Figure 18: Illustration of the human cranium.

PART 2:4 THE JOINTS

A joint is a meeting point between two bones. Some joints are free moving (articulating) joints. These are called synovial joints. The synovial joints contain free space between the bones filled with a lubricating fluid called synovial fluid. The synovial fluid prevents friction and provides a cushion to lessen the effect of shocks. In addition, the articulating surfaces of the two bones are covered with cartilage. Bursae are spaces filled with synovial fluid found wherever tendons or ligaments contact other tissues. Bursitis means inflammation of bursa. Sutures are fixed (non-moving) joints. Joints are commonly named after the articulating bones of which they are comprised. The claviculosternal joint is that between the clavicle and the sternum. The clavicle is part of the appendicular skeleton and is found in the shoulder (pectoral girdle). The sternum is the chest bone located at the middle of the anterior aspect of the thorax and is part of the axial skeleton. The tempromandibular joint is an articulation between the temporal bone of the skull and the mandible (this is the jaw joint).

PART 2:5 THE MUSCLES

Muscles are tissues made from contractile cells. They are capable of changing their shape and length, thereby creating movement. They are classified as skeletal, cardiac and smooth muscles. They can either cause locomotion of the body or movement of internal organs or body contents. For example, the contraction of cardiac muscles causes movement of blood. Smooth muscle contractions cause movements of the contents of the gastrointestinal, urinary and reproductive systems. The contraction of smooth and cardiac muscles occurs without conscious control (unconscious). These unconscious movements include peristalsis, which is the contraction of the smooth muscles in the gastrointestinal system causing the movement of food through it. The skeletal muscles are responsible for voluntary (conscious) movement, such as of the eyes, hands and legs.

PART 2:6 MUSCULOSKELETAL DISORDERS AND PROCEDURES

Arthralgia, pain in a joint, is a common symptom of many diseases like osteoarthritis, arthrochondritis, and arthritis. Ostealgia, pain in a bone, is another musculoskeletal symptom commonly associated with osteitis, osteochondritis and osteomyelitis. Arthrocentesis means medicinal removal of fluid from a joint. Surgical repair of a bone is called osteoplasty. Myoma is a benign neoplasm (cancer) of a muscle. Myositis means inflammation of a muscle. Osteomalacia is the softening of the bones, typically through a deficiency of vitamin D or calcium.

The medical term for muscles is my-. Myomalacia means softening of muscle tissue. Myospasm means continuous involuntary contraction of a muscle. Myocele means protrusion of a muscle through a tear in its outer fibrous sheet surrounding it, and myeoctomy means excision of a muscle or part of a muscle. Myalgia means pain in muscles, myositis means inflammation of a muscle or muscle group and myocarditis means inflammation of the heart muscle.

PART 2:7 REVIEW QUESTIONS

As a review, write the meaning for each of the following:

1. Osteo: _____

2. Arthro: _____

3. Chondro: _____

4. Myelo: _____

5. Myo: _____

6. Tendo: _____

7. Costo: _____

8. Myoma: _____

To exercise what you have learned, fill the blanks with the appropriate words:

1. The _____ system allows the body to move (locomote) using _____, _____ and _____ components.

2. Osteoarthritis is an inflammation of _____ and _____.

3. Osteomyelitis is inflammation of _____ and _____.

4. Myalgia means pain in _____.

5. The _____ joints contain free space between the bones filled with a lubricating fluid called synovial fluid

6. Arthrodesis is fixation of _____ by fusion.

7. _____ is the name given to the process of mineralization of the bone matrix (hardening).

8. A person who has myelitis has inflammation of the _____.

9. A person with tendonitis has an inflammation of a _____.

10. A myospasm is an involuntary contraction of a _____.

11. Fixed articulations allow no movements and include the _____ of the skull and the joints holding the teeth in position

12. Intercostal refers to the space between the _____.

CHAPTER 3

THE INTEGUMENTARY SYSTEM

Chapter Contents

PART 3:1 INTRODUCTION

The skin in the largest organ in the body and is made up of multiple layers. The skin guards the underlying muscles, bones, ligaments, nerves, and internal organs (the viscera). It protects the internal organs, contributes to heat control, and synthesizes vitamin D. Dermatology is the branch of medicine concerned with the diagnosis and treatment of skin disorders.

PART 3:2 TERMS SPECIFIC TO THE INTEGUMENTARY SYSTEM

Derma- refers to the skin, and dermis literally means the layer of connective tissue below the visible outermost layer of the skin, known as the epidermis (recall that epi- means above or upon). A person with dermatitis has an inflammation of the dermis layer of the skin. Dermatophytosis means a fungus inflammation of the skin. The dermis is connected to the epidermis by a basement membrane (a thin layer of fibers and adhesion molecules). The dermis harbors many mechanoreceptors (for perception of mechanical pressure or distortion), hair follicles, sweat glands, sebaceous glands, blood and lymphatic vessels. The sebaceous glands produce a waxy yellow body secretion called sebum. The term cutaneous denotes "of the skin." A cutaneous disease is one that attacks the skin.

PART 3:3 SKIN TISSUE

The epidermis, as you surely know by now, means the layer of tissue above the dermis, because epi- means above or upon. The epidermis is the outermost layer of the skin (Figure 19). It forms a protective layer over the body. It is made up of stratified squamous epithelium. Stratified means that it is made of multiple layers of cells, while squamous means that the cells are shaped like thin, flat plates (Figure 14, page 35). Epithelium refers to any tissue that lines body cavities and covers body surfaces (epi- "above, or on" + thelium "tissue"). The cells that make up the epidermis are Merkel cells, keratinocytes, melanocytes and Langerhans cells. Merkel cells are oval sensory cells that are responsible for perception of light touch and the discrimination of shapes and textures. There are not only found in the skin but also some parts of the mucosa, like the lips, mouth, nasal cavity and the vaginal canal. Langerhans cells are granulated dendritic cells. Dendritic cells are part of the immune system. Dendritic is an adjective that means having a branched shape resembling a tree. Langerhans cells can also be found in lymph nodes and other organs. They ingest – phagocytize – bacteria and subsequently process their antigens and display them on their cell surface. Antigens are any foreign substance that can induce an immune reaction. The first process in eliciting an immune reaction is recognizing the antigens. The Langerhans cells play an important role in capturing antigens and presenting them for other immune cells to recognize them. Melanocytes are cells that produce the dark pigment, melanin, which is responsible for the color of skin. Keratinocytes are the predominant cell type in the epidermis. They are responsible for the formation of the barrier layer against the environment. They do this partly by their ability to undergo keratinization. Keratinization allows them to become a barrier. Keratinization starts with the production of large amounts of keratin (a strong fibrous protein) and ends with the programmed cell death (apoptosis) of the keratinocytes. The now dead keratinized cells form the outermost layer, and will be constantly shed and replaced by new ones. This process is known as cornification and the outermost keratinized cells are called cornified keratinocytes. Thus, the epidermis is made of stratified squamous keratinized epithelium. The average renewal time for the epidermis is 21 days (e.g., the outermost layer of your skin gets replaced every 21 days).

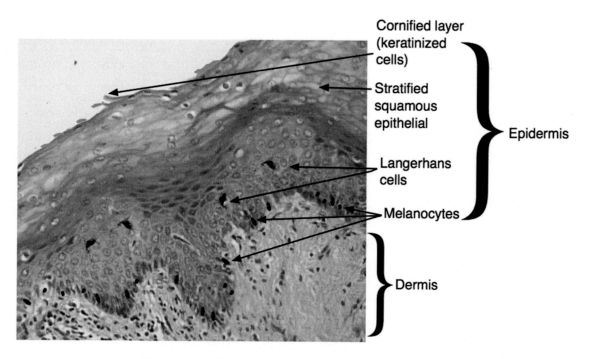

Figure 19: Microscopic illustration of human skin.

Beneath the skin there is a layer of tissue called the hypodermis (remember that hypo-means under or below). It attaches the epidermis to the underlying bone and muscle and supplies it with blood vessels, lymph vessels and nerves. It is made of connective tissue. It also contains varying amounts of subcutaneous fat. Cells types found in the hypodermis include fibroblasts, adipose cells, and macrophages. The fibroblasts produce fibers, the adipose cells store fat, and the macrophages are large immune cells that eat and ingest, phagocytize bacteria and foreign substances.

Hair follicles are invaginations of the epidermis containing different layers of cells. These cells form the matrix of the hair follicle and produce the keratin of the mature hair. The keratin producing capacity of the hair follicle is enormous, producing 0.35 mm per day.

Onycho- pertains to the nail. Onychectomy means surgical removal of nail. The nail consists of a nail plate. The plate lies in a nail groove that, like the hair follicle, is an invagination of the epidermis. Nail growth is about 0.1 mm per day. The nails, hair and the outermost layer of the skin, the keratinized epithelium, are all predominantly made of the protein keratin.

The skin also contains sebaceous glands, apocrine glands and eccrine glands. The sebaceous glands are found everywhere on the skin except on the soles and palms. They are most closely associated with hair follicles but are also common in hair-free areas like the buccal mucosa, lip, nipple, areola, labia minora and eyelids. They produce sebum, which is a bacteriostatic and fungistatic lipoidal material, and help reduce water evaporation from the skin. The scalp and the face contain up to 1000 sebaceous glands per square centimeter. Sometimes the glands become plugged with sebum, debris, and bacteria and form the blackheads and the pimples of acne. Apocrine glands are found in the axillae, genital region, breasts, external ear canal and eyelids. They do not develop until the time of puberty and consist of coiled secretary glands located in the deep dermis or subcutaneous fat and a straight duct that usually empties into a hair follicle. Their secretions may act as pheromones and are responsible for the development of body odor (pheromones are chemical substances release by an animal and affect other members of the same species). Eccrine glands are sweat glands. These are distributed everywhere on the skin surface, but their greatest concentration is found on the palms, soles and forehead. They are made of coiled glands, a coiled duct, a straight duct, an intraepidermal coil and an eccrine pore (intra "through or inside" + epi "above or upon" + dermal "pertaining to the skin"). They flood the skin surface with water for cooling.

PART 3:4 SKIN FUNCTIONS

The skin protects the body against pathogens, excessive water loss, temperature fluctuations and harmful radiation. Other functions include vitamin D synthesis and sensation. The skin also provides a site for the immune system to react with disease-causing bacteria in a manner that allows for immunity to be created.

PART 3:5 SKIN DISORDERS AND PROCEDURES

Specific disorders of the skin include pimples, papules, vesicles and pustules. A pimple is a small, hard inflamed spot on the skin. A papule is a small, raised, solid pimple or swelling (protuberance) on the skin that is typically inflamed but not producing pus. Many bacterial infections cause the formation of papules and pimples. A vesicle is a fluid-filled skin lesion. A pustule is a small blister filled with pus. Dermatitis, as you know, means inflammation of the dermis. Dermatoma refers to a skin tumor (cancer). Excessive skin, often hanging in folds, is called dermatomegaly.

The adjective cutaneous means "of the skin." Therefore, an intracutaneous test for allergy is one that uses a puncture or a prick to introduce an allergen to the skin and then looks for signs for inflammation. Transcutaneous means to measure or apply something across the depth of the skin. A neurocutaneous disorder is one that involves both the skin and the nerves.

Certain special tests are of importance in the field of dermatology. These include skin tests, fungus examinations, biopsies, and immunologic diagnosis. Skin tests include intracutaneous, scratch and patch tests. The technique of the patch test is simple, but the interpretation of it is not. For example, consider a patient presenting with dermatitis on top of the feet. It is possible that shoe leather or some chemical used in the manufacture of the leather is causing the reaction. The procedure for a patch test is to cut a 0.5 square inch piece out of the material from the inside of the shoe, moisten the material with distilled water, place it on the skin surface, and cover it with an adhesive band. Then the patch test is left on for 48 hours. When the patch test is removed, the patient is considered to have a positive patch test if there is any redness, papules, or vesiculation under the site of the testing agent. Delayed reactions to allergens can occur, and, ideally, a final reading should be made after 96 hours (4 days), that is, 2 days after the patch is removed.

Fungal examination used a simple (potassium hydroxide) KOH preparation for the detection of fungal organisms present in skin and nails. It is accomplished by scraping the diseased skin and depositing the material on a glass slide and then adding 20% aqueous KOH solution and a coverslip. The slide is then examined microscopically for fungal organisms. The species of fungus obtained can then be identified based on its morphology.

PART 3:6 REVIEW QUESTIONS

As a review, write the meaning for each of the following:

1. Dermis: _____
2. Epidermis: _____
3. Subcutaneous: _____
4. Onycho: _____
5. Sebaceous: _____
6. Melanocyte: _____
7. Dendritic: _____
8. Cornification: _____
9. Squamous: _____
10. Transcutaneous:_____
11. Intraepidermal: _____
12. Pimples: _____
13. Papules: _____
14. Vesicles:_____
15. Pustules:_____

To exercise what you have learned, fill the blanks with the appropriate words:

1. A person with dermatophytosis has a fungal infection of the _____.
2. Onychectomy is the surgical removal of the _____ of a finger or a toe.
3. An introduction of an allergen into the skin is called _____.
4. _____ means to measure or apply something across the depth of the skin. _____ test for allergy uses a puncture or a prick to introduce an allergen to the skin and then looks for signs for inflammation.
5. The subcutaneous fat is found in the _____.

CHAPTER 4

THE RESPIRATORY SYSTEM

Chapter Contents

PART 4:1 INTRODUCTION

The respiratory system includes the lungs, pleura, bronchi, trachea, larynx, pharynx, tonsils and nose. The respiratory system is divided into the upper and lower respiratory systems. The upper respiratory system is comprised of the nose, pharynx and tonsils. The lower respiratory system is made of the larynx, trachea, bronchi, pleura and the lungs. The lungs contain the secondary and tertiary bronchi, the bronchioles, and alveoli.

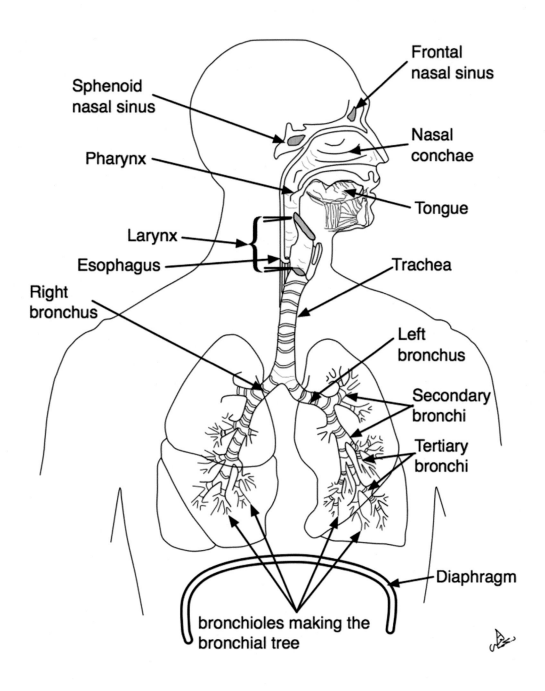

Figure 20: Illustration of the human respiratory system.

PART 4:2 TERMS SPECIFIC TO THE RESPIRATORY SYSTEM

The terms used for the nose include nas- and rhino-. A person with an inflammation of the nose, due, for example, to influenza, in medical terms is said to suffer from rhinitis. The cavity of the nose is called the nasal cavity. A group of viruses that can infect the nasal cavity are called rhinoviruses. The nasal sinuses are air-filled cavities in the cranium bones lined with mucus membranes. The air passes through the nasal cavity, which contains nasal conchae (turbinates). The function of the nasal conchae is to filter and humidify the incoming air. That is, the conchae are responsible for circulating the air against the nasal mucosa in order to filter and humidify it. The conchae are long, narrow, curled bone shelves that protrude into the breathing passage of the nose dividing the nasal airway into four groove-like air passages.

Laryng- denotes the larynx (colloquially called the "voice box"). A laryngoscope is the instrument used for the examination of the larynx. Trache- stands for the upper windpipe or trachea. A person with tracheitis has inflammation of the trachea. Bronch- is the root for the lower windpipe or bronchus, which is the airway leading from the end of the trachea to the lung. There are two bronchi, each leading to one lung. Bronchitis means inflammation of the bronchi. The small brunches of the bronchi, inside the lungs, are called bronchioles.

Pulmon(o)- and pneum(o, on)- are stems for lung. The pulmonary blood circulation refers to the blood circulation to the lungs. Pneumonia refers to an inflammation of the lungs with consolidation and exudation caused by bacterial infection (mainly the bacterial species *Streptococcus pneumoniae*), but viruses and (rarely) fungi can also cause pneumonia. Pneumonitis is a general term that refers to inflammation of the lungs. Pneum(o, on)- can also be used to refer to air. For example, pneumothorax refers to a condition in which air escapes the lungs and finds its way to the thoracic cavity.

-pnea and pneo- both stands for breathing. Pneodynamics is the mechanism of breathing. Recall that the prefix a- means without or cessation of. Thus, apnea means a temporary cessation of breathing. Similarly, remembering that the prefix dys- means bad, difficult or painful, dyspnea means difficult and painful breathing. Orthopnea (ortho "straight" + pnea "breathing") is shortness of breath (dyspnea), which occurs when lying flat, causing a person to have to sleep propped up in bed or sitting on a chair. It is the opposite of platypnea.

PART 4:3 TISSUES

The lining of the nasal cavity and the respiratory airways (except for the pharynx, terminal bronchioles and alveoli) is made of pseudostratified columnar ciliated respiratory epithelium with goblet cells. The tissue is called pseudostratified (pseudo "false" + stratified "layered") because it appears layered when in fact all the cells rest on the same basement membrane (Figure 14, page 35). This is the case because some cells are longer and thus extend from the basement membrane to the outermost surface while other cells are shorter, causing the tissue to appear stratified. That is because the nuclei in the cells appear to form multiple layers (Figure 21) giving the illusion of stratification. Goblet means bowl-shaped, and goblet cells are bowl-shaped cells that produce protective mucus to cover the epithelial surface and trap bacteria and particulates. The cilia are tiny projections that beat rhythmically to move the mucus and any attached bacteria or particulates, such as dust, out of the body through the cough reflex (Figure 21).

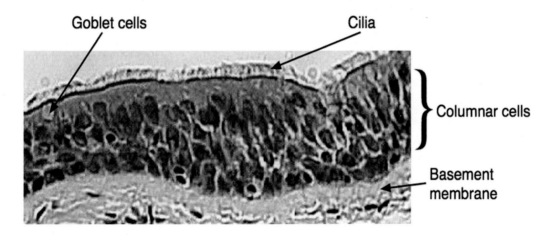

Figure 21: Microscopic image of the pseudostratified columnar ciliated respiratory epithelium with goblet cells.

The air flows through the nasal cavity, pharynx, larynx, and trachea and is then divided between the left and right bronchi. From there the air enters the lungs and is distributed through the secondary and tertiary bronchi and finally through the bronchioles into the terminal (respiratory) bronchioles, which empty their air into the alveolar ducts and finally the alveoli (singular alveolus). Each alveolus is a hollow cavity made of the following types of pneumocytes: (1) type I cells (squamous alveolar cells) that form the alveolar wall; (2) type II cells (great granular alveolar cells), which produce pulmonary surfactant to lower the surface tension of water and allow the alveoli to inflate; and (3) macrophages that destroy foreign materials such as bacteria. Typically, the lungs contain 700 million alveoli producing 70 m^2 of surface area. Each alveolus is wrapped in a fine mesh of capillaries called a capillary bed

(Figure 22). The alveoli represent the major site where gases are exchanged, allowing for the blood to get oxygenated (e.g., oxygen enters to blood and carbon dioxide leaves).

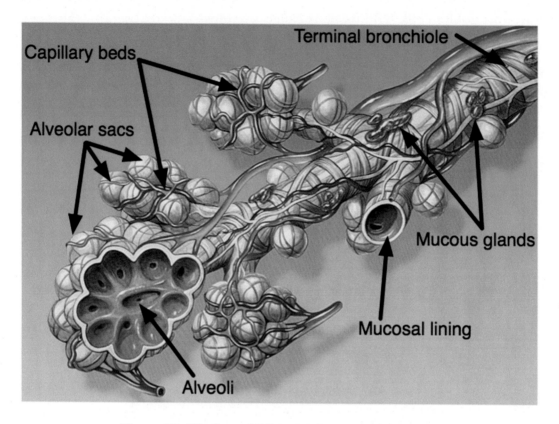

Figure 22: The bronchioles and the alveoli structure.
Obtained from Patrick J. Lunch under Creative Common Attribution 2.5 License, 2006.

PART 4:4 FUNCTIONS

Functions of the respiratory system include: gas exchange, vocalization, temperature control, some metabolic and endocrine functions, and defense. Gas exchange is mediated by ventilation. Ventilation consists of inhalation and exhalation. Inhalation, intake of air through the nose or mouth to the lungs, is initiated by the diaphragm and, to a lesser extent, the external intercostal muscles. Normal resting respirations are 10 to 18 breaths per minute. When the diaphragm and external intercostals contract, the ribcage (thoracic cavity) expands, creating a negative pressure inside the lungs with respect to the atmospheric pressure, forcing air to enter into the lungs. Exhalation, the act of breathing air out, is normally a passive process; nonetheless, active forced exhalation is achieved in certain circumstances by the abdominal and internal intercostal muscles contracting and diminishing the volume of the ribcage, thus increasing its pressure and forcing air out. This happens, for instance, in coughing and sneezing. Gas exchange is the major function of the lungs. This exchange facilitates oxygenation of the blood with a simultaneous removal of carbon dioxide from the circulation. Gas exchange occurs in the alveoli.

Vocalization means producing noises to express feelings and thoughts. The movement of air through the larynx, pharynx and mouth allows humans to speak, or phonate. The vibration of air through the larynx, which contains the vocal chords, in humans allow for singing and vocalization. Air movement is vital for communication in humans

In addition to the functions of gas exchange and vocalization, the lungs have a number of metabolic functions and also help cool the body. The respiratory system helps reduce body temperature by increasing ventilation through the exhalation of warm air. The lungs produce surfactant for local use and fibrinolytic enzymes that help dissolve blood clots. The lungs also activate one hormone: the physiologically inactive decapeptide angiotensin I is converted to the pressor, aldosterone-stimulating octapeptide angiotensin II in the pulmonary circulation via a converting enzyme. The reaction occurs in other tissues as well, but it is particularly prominent in the lungs. The converting enzyme also inactivates bradykinin, and the end result is control of blood pressure.

Airway epithelial cells can secrete a variety of molecules that aid in lung defense. Secretory immunoglobulins (IgA), collectins (including surfactant A and D), defensins and other peptides and proteases, reactive oxygen species, and reactive nitrogen species are all generated by airway epithelial cells. These secretions can act directly as antimicrobials to help keep the airway free of infection.

PART 4:5 DISORDERS AND PROCEDURES

Bronchoscopy is a test to view the airways and diagnose lung diseases. A bronchoscope, a devise used to see the inside of the airways, is used in bronchoscopy. Note that the suffix for breathing is -pnea and recall that the prefix a- means without or cessation of. Therefore, apnea refers to a temporary cessation of breathing, especially during sleeping. Many people suffer from sleep apnea, especially obese individuals. Similarly, remember that the prefix dys- means bad, difficult or painful. Therefore, dyspnea means difficult, painful breathing. Pharyngitis means inflammation of the pharynx (the throat). Emphysema, from Greek, meaning to puff up, is a serious disease characterized by the destruction of the gas-exchanging airspaces (e.g., the respiratory bronchioles, alveolar ducts and alveoli). Their walls are destroyed, forcing the airspaces to join together into abnormal and much larger airspaces (Figure 23). Emphysema causes chronic sever dyspnea, and smoking is the main cause of it.

Bronchopneumonia is a patchy consolidation involving one or several lobes. Bronchitis means inflammation of the bronchial tree. Bronchorrhea is the production of excessive amounts of watery sputum (-rrhea is the suffix for excessive discharge of flow). Bronchospasm is a sudden construction of the muscles in the walls of the bronchioles causing difficulty in breathing (dyspnea). Bronchostenosis refers to chronic narrowing (-stenosis) of the bronchi. Since the stem for the nose is rhino-, rhinitis means inflammation of the nasal cavity, while rhinalgia or rhinodynia refer to pain in the nose. Rhinorrhea is the production of excessive nasal mucus discharge. Rhinoplasty refers to a procedure in plastic surgery in which the structure of the nose is changed. A rhinoscope (or nasoscope) is a thin tube-like instrument used to examine the inside of the nose in the procedure known as rhinoscopy. Rhinostenosis means narrowing of the passages of the nasal cavity, sinusitis is inflammation of the nasal sinuses, and tracheomegaly is an abnormally enlarged (dilated) trachea, which may result from infection or prolonged positive pressure ventilation. Recall that -megaly means enlargement.

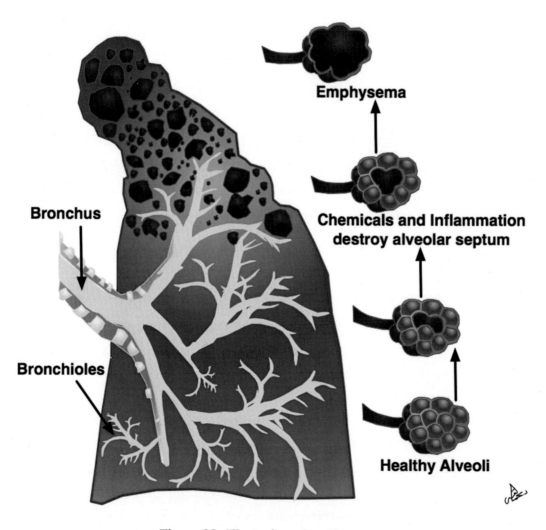

Figure 23: Illustraion of emphysema.

PART 4:6 REVIEW QUESTIONS

As a review, write the meaning for each of the following:

1. Rhino: _____
2. Naso: _____
3. Laryngo: _____
4. Tracheo: _____
5. Broncho: _____
6. Pulmo: _____
7. Pneumo: _____
8. Bronchospasm: _____
9. Bronchorrhea: _____
10. Pneo: _____

To exercise what you have learned, fill the blanks with the appropriate words:

1. A patient with rhinitis has an _____.
2. A laryngoscopy is an examination of the _____.
3. Tracheitis is the inflammation of _____.
4. A student who has bronchitis has an inflammation of the _____.
5. The pulmonary artery leads to the _____.
6. An inflammation of the lungs with consolidation is called _____.
7. _____ is a patchy consolidation involving one or several lobes.
8. _____ is the production of excessive amounts of watery sputum.
9. _____ is a sudden construction of the muscles in the walls of the bronchioles causing difficulty in breathing (dyspnea).
10. The tissue is called _____ because it appears layered when in fact all the cells rest on the same basement membrane.
11. _____, from Greek, meaning to puff up, is a serious disease characterized by the destruction of the gas-exchanging airspaces.
12. _____ refers to a procedure in plastic surgery in which the structure of the nose is changed.
13. A _____ is a thin tube-like instrument used to examine the inside of the nose in the procedure known as rhinoscopy.
14. _____ means narrowing of the passages of the nasal cavity.
15. _____ is inflammation of the nasal sinuses.
16. _____ means producing noises to express feelings and thoughts.
17. Ventilation consists of _____ and _____.
18. _____ means a temporary cessation of breathing.

19. Pneodynamics is the mechanism of _____.

20. _____ is a patchy consolidation involving one or several lobes.

21. _____ means inflammation of the bronchial tree.

22. _____ is the production of excessive amounts of watery sputum by the bronchi.

23. _____ is a sudden construction of the muscles in the walls of the bronchioles causing difficulty in breathing (_____).

24. _____ refers to chronic narrowing of a bronchus.

25. _____ means inflammation of the nasal cavity.

26. _____or _____ refer to pain in the nose.

Describe the respiratory epithelium structure and function.

_____

_____

_____

_____

_____

List the organs air passes through from the atmosphere to the blood.

_____

_____

_____

_____

_____

Define emphysema and list its symptoms.

_____

_____

_____

_____

CHAPTER 5

THE DIGESTIVE SYSTEM

Chapter Contents

PART 5:1 INTRODUCTION

The digestive system begins at the mouth, where food enters, and ends at the anus, where solid wastes (feces or stool) leave the body. The digestive tract consists of the oral cavity, pharynx, esophagus, stomach, small intestine, large intestine, rectum and anus. The small intestine is divided into the duodenum, jejunum, and ileum. The large intestine is divided into the cecum, vermiform appendix, colon, rectum and anus. Other accessory organs of the digestive system are the teeth, tongue, salivary glands, gallbladder, liver and pancreas. The digestive system is also called the gastrointestinal tract (GI tract) and the alimentary canal. The part of the alimentary canal below the stomach is commonly called the bowels.

PART 5:2 TERMS SPECIFIC TO THE DIGESTIVE SYSTEM

One medical term referring to the mouth is -stoma-. Stomatitis is inflammation of the mouth and xerostomia is a condition characterized by a pathologically dry mouth. The mouth is also called the buccal cavity or the oral cavity. The month consists of the lips anteriorly, the cheeks laterally, the tongue and its muscles inferiorly, and the hard and soft palate superiorly. The palate forms the roof of the mouth. The hard palate is the bony anterior portion of the palate that is covered with mucous membrane. The soft palate is the flexible posterior portion of the palate. It has the important role of closing the nasal passage during swallowing to prevent food and liquid from moving upward into the nasal cavity. The uvula hangs from the posterior free edge of the soft palate (Figure 24). It plays a role in the formation of some speech sounds. Other structures of the mouth include the tongue, salivary glands, teeth, gums and the periodontium.

Lingua- and gloss- are the terms used for the tongue. Bilingual refers to the ability to speak two languages. The tongue is made of voluntary skeletal muscles covered with a mucous membrane. The tongue changes size, shape and location to help position food during mastication (chewing). Tongue muscles are either intrinsic, for size and shape control, or extrinsic, such as the genioglossus (to stick the tongue outside) and the hyoglossus (to depresses the tongue). The upper surface of the tongue is called the dorsum. This surface has tough protective covering and, in some areas, small bumps called papillae (singular, papilla), which contain the taste buds. The sublingual surface of the tongue, and the tissues located under the tongue, are covered with delicate highly vascular tissue (e.g., containing many blood vessels). The term sublingual means under the tongue. It is worth noting that some drugs can be administered sublingually where they can be quickly absorbed into the bloodstream.

The lingual fernum attaches the tongue to the floor of the mouth and limit its motion. The lips, also known as labia, form the opening to the oral cavity (singular, labium). The lips are where the skin continues into the gastrointestinal tract and changes into a mucous membrane. The boundary between the two is sensitive. Cheil- is the stem designating the lips. The upper and lower labial frenum are narrow bands of tissue that attach the lips to the jaws (Figure 24).

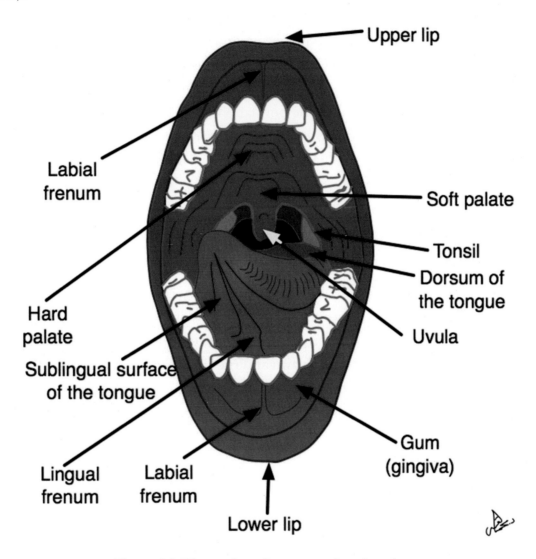

Figure 24: Illustration of tongue and oral cavity.

Dent- and odont- are the terms for teeth. Dentition refers to the natural teeth arranged in the upper and lower jaws. Orthodontist is the name given to the medical practitioner responsible for treating irregularities in the teeth and jaws, usually by using braces. Dentistry is the medical science concerned with the prevention and treatment of teeth and gum disorders and diseases, requiring graduation from a dental school. Graduates from dentistry schools are called dentists.

Gingiv- refers to the gums, which is the mucous membrane that surrounds the teeth, covers the bone of the dental arches and lines the cheeks. Gingivitis means inflammation of the gums. The dental arches are the bony structures of the oral cavity (the maxillary and mandibular arches). These structures, commonly called the upper and lower jaws, firmly hold the teeth in position. The periodontium (peri "surrounding" + odonti "teeth" + ium "tissue") consist of the bone and soft tissues that surround and support the teeth. The human dentition (arrangement and types of teeth) includes four types of teeth: incisors and canines (also known as cuspids) that are used for biting and tearing, plus premolars (also known as bicuspids) and molars that are used for chewing and grinding. The primary dentition, also known as the deciduous dentition or baby teeth, consists of 20 teeth that are normally lost during childhood and are replaced by the permanent teeth. These deciduous teeth include: 8 incisors, 4 canines, 8 molars, and no premolars. The permanent dentition consists of 32 teeth that are designed to last a lifetime. These teeth include: 8 incisors, 4 canines, 8 premolars, and 12 molars. Edentulous means without teeth, and describes the situation of having lost natural permanent teeth. In dentistry, occlusion describes any contact between the chewing surfaces of the upper and lower teeth. Malocclusion is any deviation from the normal positioning of the upper teeth against the lower teeth (recall that the prefix mal- means bad).

The crown is the portion of a tooth that is visible. It is covered with enamel, which is the hardest substance in the body. The roots of the tooth hold it securely in place within the dental arch. The root is protected by cementum, which is strong, but not as hard as enamel. The cervix (neck) of the tooth is where the crown and root meets. Dentin makes up the bulk of the tooth structure and is protected on the outer surfaces by the enamel and cementum (Figure 25). The pulp consists of a rich supply of blood vessels and nerves that provide nutrients and innervation to the tooth. In the crown, the pulp is located in the pulp cavity. In the root, the pulp continues through the root canal.

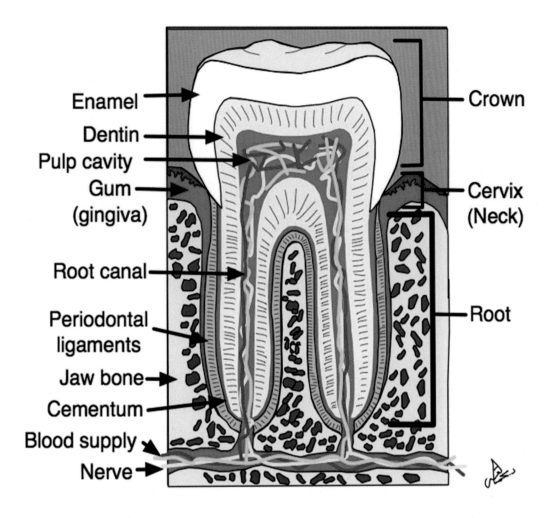

Figure 25: Illustration of the structures and tissues of the tooth.

Saliva is a colorless liquid that moistens the mouth, begins the digestive process, and lubricates food during chewing and swallowing. There are three pairs of salivary glands, which secrete saliva that is carried by ducts into the mouth. The parotid glands are located slightly below and in front of the ears. The ducts for these glands are on the inside of the cheek near the upper molars. The sublingual glands and their ducts are located on the floor of the mouth under the tongue. The submandibular glands and their ducts are located on the floor of the mouth.

Food and liquids pass from the mouth to the pharynx, which is a common passageway for both air and food. The epiglottis, part of the larynx, is a lid-like structure that closes off the entrance of the trachea (windpipe) to prevent food and liquid from moving from the pharynx to the trachea. From the pharynx, food and liquid move down a muscular tube called the esophagus. The lower esophageal sphincter, called the cardiac sphincter (because it is located near the heart) or the gastroesophageal sphincter (because it is also located between the stomach and the esophagus), prevents food and liquid from returning to the esophagus from the stomach. A sphincter is a muscular ring that controls the flow within a tube. This sphincter normally opens to allow the flow of food and liquid into the stomach and closes to prevent the stomach contents from regurgitating into the esophagus (regurgitate means to flow backward).

Gastr- signifies the stomach. The stomach is a sac-like organ composed of the fundus (upper, rounded part), body (main portion), and antrum (lower part). Rugae are folds in the mucosa lining the stomach. Glands located within these folds produce gastric juices, which aid in digestion, and mucus secretion, which creates a protective coating on the lining of the stomach. The pylorus is the narrow passage that connects the stomach with the small intestine. Pylorus, from Greek, means gatekeeper. The pyloric sphincter is the ring-like muscle that controls the flow from the stomach to the duodenum of the small intestine.

Enter- means the small intestine and gastr- means the stomach, so gastroenteritis means inflammation of the stomach and the small intestine. Duoden- means the duodenum, which is the first part of the small intestine. A duodenal ulcer, for example, is an ulcer located in the duodenum. Jejun- pertains to the jejunum, which is the second part of the small intestine. A jejunostomy refers to an artificial opening into the jejunum. Ile- means the ileum, which is the third and last part of the small intestine. Ileitis means inflammation of the ileum. The ileocecal valve is the valve between the ileum and the cecum. The cecum is the first part of the large intestine.

The major parts of the large intestine are the cecum, colon, rectum, vermiform appendix and anus. The cecum is a pouch that lies on the right side of the abdomen. It extends from the end of the ileum to the beginning of the colon. The vermiform appendix, commonly called the appendix, hangs from the lower portion of the cecum. The term vermiform refers to a worm-like shape. The appendix contains lymphoid tissue and may play an immune function. Col- is the term for the colon. The colon is subdivided into four parts: the ascending colon (ascending means moving upward), the transverse colon (transverse means moving across), descending colon (descending means moving downwards) and the sigmoid colon (sigmoid means like the letter S).

Procto- and ano- are the roots used for the rectum and anus, respectively. Proctitis is an inflammation of the rectum. The rectum, which is the widest division of the large intestine, makes up the last 4 inches of it and ends at the anus. The anus is the lower opening of the digestive tract. The internal and external anal sphincters control the flow of waste through the anus.

The term hepat- refers to the liver. Hepatocytes are liver cells. Hepatitis means inflammation of the liver. The liver has important functions, including detoxifying blood (removing toxins) and converting food into the fuel and nutrients needed by the body. For example, the liver removes excessive blood glucose and stores it as glycogen (starch). Then the liver converts glycogen back to glucose and releases it between meals. This is controlled by the hormones insulin and glucagon. The liver also destroys old erythrocytes (red blood cells), removes toxins from the blood, and manufactures some blood proteins. Bilirubin, which is the pigment produced from the breakdown of hemoglobin, is released by the liver in bile. Bile, which aids in the digestion of lipids and fats, is a digestive juice secreted by the liver. Bile travels from the liver to the gallbladder, where it is concentrated and stored. The biliary tree provides the channels through which bile is transported from the liver to the small intestine. Biliary means pertaining to bile. Small ducts in the liver join together to form the biliary tree. The trunk of the tree, which is just outside the liver, is known as the common hepatic bile duct. The bile travels from the liver through the common hepatic duct to the gallbladder through a narrow duct called the cystic duct. The cystic duct not only carries bile to the gallbladder from the common hepatic duct, but also moves the bile back to it. This is because the common hepatic duct joins the pancreatic duct, and together they open into the duodenum of the small intestine. Cholecyst- refers to the gallbladder. The gallbladder is a pear-shaped organ about the size of an egg located under the liver. The gallbladder stores and concentrates the bile for later use. The pancreas is a soft gland located behind the stomach, which produces pancreatic juices. These juices contain hydrolytic (digestive) enzymes for the digestion of foodstuff and sodium bicarbonate that aids in the neutralization of stomach acids. The pancreas also controls blood glucose concentration via the production of two hormones: insulin and glucagon. Insulin makes the liver and other body organs absorb glucose, thus reducing blood glucose concentration, while glucagon brings about the release of glucose from the liver to increase blood glucose concentration.

PART 5:3 TISSUES

The entire gastrointestinal tract has some important common structural characteristics. That is, it is a hollow tube with a lumen made up of four main layers: the mucosa, submucosa, muscularis and serosa. The lining of the gastrointestinal tract is made of epithelial cells. The lining of the oral cavity, pharynx, esophagus, rectum and the anus is made of stratified squamous epithelium. The lining of the small intestine is made of simple columnar epithelium (Figure 14, page 35).

PART 5:4 FUNCTIONS

Food is digested into simple nutrients. The first step in digestion is mastication, also called chewing, which is the process of the mechanical breakdown of food into small pieces, mixing it with saliva and preparing it for swallowing as a bolus (a mass of food that has been chewed and is ready for swallowing). Swallowing is the passage of food from the mouth, pharynx and esophagus to the stomach. Food moves through the esophagus and the GI tract through peristalsis, which is a series of wave-like contractions of the smooth muscles in a single direction. In the stomach food is converted into chyme (pronounced kym), which is a semifluid mass of partly digested food. In the intestine the chyme is mixed with bile and pancreatic juices. The bile makes the fat globules smaller and more water-soluble. This action of bile is called emulsification (to make an emulsion of fat, which is a fine dispersion of very small droplets of fat in liquid). Carbohydrates are digested into simple sugars, fats are digested into fatty acids and glycerol, and proteins are digested into amino acids. In addition to these nutrients the body needs small amounts of vitamins and minerals. Absorption is the transport of the completely digested nutrients into the bloodstream for distribution to all body cells. The mucosa of the small intestine, where most of the adsorption takes place, is covered with finger-like projections called villi (singular, vilus), which increase the surface area of absorption. Each vilus contains blood vessels and lacteals. Lacteals are specialized lymphatic vessels, which absorb fats and fat-soluble vitamins. At the end of the digestion and adsorption process, feces, also called stool, are the remaining solid wastes formed in the large intestine and stored in the sigmoid colon and rectum. Emptying the large intestine is called defecation. Flatulence, also called flatus, is the passage of gases through the anus. Bacteria are responsible for the production of these gases.

PART 5:5 DISORDERS AND PROCEDURES

Stomatitis is an inflammation of the mouth and xerostomia is a condition characterized by a pathologically dry mouth. Xerostomia can be induced by smoking. Gingivitis means inflammation of the gums. Gingivitis commonly develops due to smoking and poor oral hygiene. Glossitis means inflammation of the tongue. Some bacteria, viruses and fungi are known to cause glossitis. Cheiloplasty refers to surgical repair of the lips (plastic surgery). Dentalgia means tooth pain. Gastritis is an inflammation of the stomach. Enterocolitis means inflammation of the small and large intestine. Ileitis means inflammation of the ileum. Proctitis is an inflammation of the rectum.

Colostomy is a surgical procedure in which an artificial opening into the colon is created. Cholecystectomy is the name given to the surgical procedure for the removal of the gallbladder. Gastrectomy is the surgical removal of the stomach. The root, lapar- and abdomin-, mean abdomen. Laparoscopy is a surgical procedure in which a fiber-optic instrument in inserted through the abdominal wall to view the organs in the abdomen and operate on them surgically. An anoscopy is the visual examination of the anal canal and lower rectum. An anoscope, which is a short speculum, is used for this procedure. A speculum is an instrument used to enlarge the opening of any body cavity to facilitate inspection of its interior. An esophagogastroduodenoscopy is an endoscopic procedure that allows direct visualization of the upper GI tract, which includes the esophagus, stomach, and upper duodenum.

Diarrhea and constipation are two very common symptoms of gastrointestinal diseases. Diarrhea is a condition in which feces are discharged from the bowels frequently and in a liquid form. Constipation is a condition in which there is difficulty in emptying the bowels, usually associated with hardened feces.

There are many bacteria living inside the gastrointestinal system. Most of these bacteria are essential for the normal digestion and absorption. They also produce many vitamins and prevent the colonization of harmful pathogens. These good bacteria are called probiotics. If they are killed, due to antibiotics administration for example, antibiotics associated diarrhea or pseudomembranous colitis can develop. A fecal occult blood test is a laboratory test for hidden blood in feces. A hemorrhoidectomy is the surgical removal of hemorrhoids (hemorrhoid means piles, and -ectomy means surgical removal).

PART 5:6 REVIEW QUESTIONS

As a review, write the meaning for each of the following:

1. Stoma: _____

2. Lingual/glossa: _____

3. Dento/odonto: _____

4. Cheilo: _____

5. Gingivo: _____

6. Gastro: _____

7. Duodeno: _____

8. Jejuno: _____

9. Ileo: _____

10. Entero: _____

11. Colo: _____

12. Procto: _____

13. Ano: _____

14. Hepato: _____

15. Cholecysto: _____

16. Laparo: _____

17. Dentalgia: _____

18. Diarrhea: _____

19. Constipation:_____

20. Probiotic bacteria: _____

To exercise what you have learned, fill the blanks with the appropriate words:

1. A person with xerostomia has _____.

2. Stomatitis refers to _____.

3. Bilingual refers to the ability to speak two _____.

4. A cheiloplasty is the surgical repair of a defect in the _____.

5. Gingivitis means inflammation of the _____.

6. Gastroenteritis is an inflammation of the _____ and the _____.

7. A duodenal ulcer is an ulcer located at _____.

8. Ileitis means _____ of the _____.

9. Inflammation of the liver is called _____.

10. Cholecystectomy refers to the surgical removal of the _____.

11. During laparoscopic surgery a fiber-optic pass through the _____.

List the parts where food must pass through from the mouth to the anus.

_____

_____

_____

_____

_____

Name one cause for antibiotic-associated diarrhea.

_____

CHAPTER 6

THE CARDIOVASCULAR SYSTEM

Chapter Contents

PART 6:1 INTRODUCTION

The term cardiovascular refers to the heart and blood vessels (cardio "heart" + vascul "blood vessels" + -ar "pertaining to"). The blood vessels are divided into arteries, veins and capillaries. The arteries carry blood away from the heart. The veins carry blood toward the heart. The capillaries are very narrow vessels that allow for the blood to reach the tissues and the cells. The main function of the cardiovascular system is the transportation to gases (oxygen and carbon dioxide), nutrients, wastes and hormones. In addition, the cardiovascular system, also named the circulatory system, helps in stabilizing body temperature, pH and fight diseases. The heart is divided into chambers. These chambers are the atria (singular, atrium) and the ventricles. The atria are the upper chambers of the heart. The atria receive all the blood vessels incoming to the heart. The left and right atria are separated by the interatrial septum, which is a wall that separates the two atria (recall that inter- means between). The ventricles are the two lower chambers of the heart. They are the pumping chambers of the heart. Thus, all the blood vessels carrying outgoing blood for the heart emerge from the ventricles. The ventricles of the heart are separated by an interventricular septum. The walls of the ventricles are thicker than those of the atria because they must pump blood throughout the whole body (Figure 26).

The valves of the heart control the blood flow within heart. There are four valves: the tricuspid, pulmonary semilunar, mitral, and aortic semilunar valves (Figure 26). If any of these valves is malfunctioning, blood does not flow properly through the heart and cannot be pumped effectively to all parts of the body. The tricuspid valve controls the opening between the right atrium and the right ventricle. Tricuspid means having three cusps (points). The pulmonary semilunar valve is located between the right ventricle and the pulmonary artery. Pulmonary means pertaining to the lungs, and semilunar means half-moon – this valve is shaped like a half-moon. The mitral valve, also called the bicuspid valve, is located between the left atrium and the left ventricle. Mitral means shaped like a bishop's miter (hat). Bicuspid means having two cusps. The aortic semilunar valve is located between the left ventricle and the aorta (Figure 26).

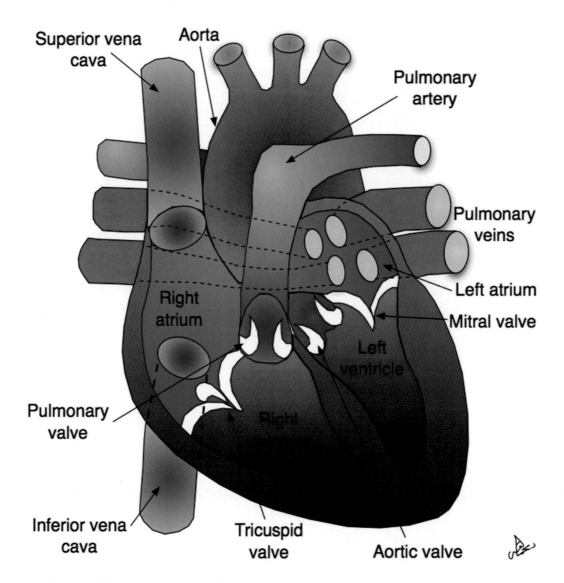

Figure 26: Illustration of the heart chambers, valves and major blood vessels.

PART 6:2 TERMS SPECIFIC TO THE CARDIOVASCULAR SYSTEM

Table 10 lists some of the most common roots, suffixes and prefixes used to describe the cardiovascular system. For example, the term cardi- means heart. Thus, an electrocardiogram (ECG) is a visual record (gram) of the heart's electrical activity. This visual recording of the heart electrical activity is made using an instrument called an electrocardiograph. On the other hand, the instrument called an echocardiograph is used for making a visual record of the sound waves of the heart (note that echo- means sound). Importantly, the term myocardial infarction (MI) is commonly used to refer to the death of part of the heart muscle (recall that myo- means muscle). Myocardial infarction, also known as heart attack, results from the interruption of blood supply to a part of the heart muscle, causing this part of the heart muscle to die. The interruption of the blood supply is most commonly due to an arteriosclerotic lesion in a coronary artery. Arteriosclerosis is a disease characterized by the deposition of a plaque of fatty material on the inner walls of the arteries. The coronary arteries are the ones that supply blood to the heart muscle. Myocardial infraction, abbreviated MI, is a very common medical condition in modern society and leads to many deaths worldwide.

The terms haem-, hem-, hemato- and -aemia mean blood. Thus, hemorrhage means bleeding and hemolysis means breakdown of blood cells (note that -rrhagia is a suffix meaning excessive flow and -lysis means breakdown). Bacteraemia, viraemia and toxemia mean the presence of bacteria, viruses and toxins in the blood, respectively. Similarly, hyperglycemia, hyperuricemia and hyperprolactinemia mean an increase in the concentration of glucose, uric acid and the hormone prolactin in the blood, respectively.

The average adult has a blood volume of approximately 5 liter, which is composed of plasma and several formed elements (cells). About 55% of blood is plasma, a fluid that circulates many substances such as electrolytes, proteins, sugars, amino acids, fatty acids, urea, lactate and hormones. The formed elements of blood include erythrocytes (red blood cells), leukocytes (white blood cells) and thrombocytes (platelets). Erythrocytes are important for the transportation of oxygen. Leukocytes help protects the body against bacteria, viruses and parasites. Thrombocytes are important for blood clotting (thrombosis). The term thromb- means blood clot. Thrombosis is the process of blood clotting. A mobile blood clot that may occlude arteries or veins is called a thrombus.

Recall that the term -penia means deficiency. Therefore, thrombocytopenia and leuckopenia mean a low level of thrombocytes and leukocytes, respectively. Plasma also contains the clotting factors. If the clotting factors are removed from the plasma, the remaining fluid is called serum. The study of serum is called serology. Serum is used in many diagnostic tests, and in blood typing. Blood is centrifuged to remove the formed elements. Anti-coagulated blood yields plasma while coagulated blood, where the clotting factors were consumed by coagulation, yields serum.

Vas- means vessel. Therefore, vasospasm means the contraction of blood vessels, which causes a reduction in blood flow (note that spasm means involuntary contraction). Angi- also means vessel. Angiitis, like vasculitis, means inflammation of blood vessels. Phleb- means vein. Thrombophlebitis means vein inflammation associated with blood clotting (thrombosis) inside the vein.

Table 10: List of terms used to describe the cardiovascular

Term	Meaning	Example
Cardio-	Heart	Echocardiogram: sound wave image of the heart
Haem-	Blood	Haematoma: a tumor or swelling filled with blood
Thromb-	Clot	Thrombocytopenia: deficiency of thrombocytes in blood
Ethro-	Red	Erythrocyte: red blood cell
Leuko-	White	Leukocyte: white blood cell
-aemia	Blood	Bacteremia: presence of bacteria in blood
Vas-	Vessel	Cerebrovascular: the blood vessels of the cerebrum of the brain
-penia	Deficiency	Leukocytopenia: low level of leukocytes
Angi-	Vessel	Angiogenesis: growth of blood vessels
Arteri-	Artery	Arteritis: inflammation of arteries
Phleb-	Vein	Phlebitis: inflammation of veins

PART 6:3 TISSUES

Cardi-, as stated previously, is the medical stem for the heart. The heart is a hollow, muscular organ located between the lungs and is enclosed inside a sac. This sac is called the pericardium, also called the pericardial sac, which is a fibrous membrane that forms a sac surrounding the heart (recall that peri- means surrounding). This sac is made of two layers, one free and the other attached to the myocardium. The free layer, the parietal pericardium, is the tough outer layer of the pericardium, which protects the heart. The second layer, the visceral pericardium, is the inner layer of the pericardium that forms the outer layer of the heart organ. That is, the visceral pericardium is attached to the myocardium (Figure 27). When the visceral pericardium is referred to as the outer layer of the heart, it is then called the epicardium (recall that epi- mean above, upon or on). Pericardial fluid is found between these two layers of the pericardium. The pericardial fluid acts as a lubricant to prevent friction when the heart beats. The walls of the heart are made of three layers. From outside to inside, these are the epicardium, the myocardium and the endocardium. The epicardium is the external layer of the heart and is the same as the visceral pericardium, as stated above. The myocardium is the middle thick layer of the heart. It is made of specialized muscles cells called cardiac muscle cells. The endocardium, the innermost layer of the heart, consists of an epithelium tissue that lines the inside of the heart chambers (endo- "within" + cardium "heart tissue"). The endocardium is the surface that comes into contact with the blood.

The myocardium, which beats constantly, must have a continuous supply of oxygen and nutrients plus rapid waste removal to survive. Oxygen-rich blood is supplied via the coronary arteries and the oxygen-poor blood, along with wastes and carbon dioxide, are removed via the coronary veins. The coronary arteries are prone to arteriosclerosis (arterio "aretery" + sclerosis "hardening and narrowing"), which is caused due to the accumulation of fatty material (such as cholesterol) in the walls of the arteries. This leads to inadequate blood supply to the myocardium, which is a dangerous condition called ischemia. If the condition is not treated the heart may suffer from a myocardial infraction. Myocardial infraction, commonly known as a heart attack, is the death of part of the myocardium. Symptoms of myocardial infraction include retrosternal pain (chest pain originating from behind the sternum – recall that retro- means behind and the sternum is the breastbone). Other symptoms include shortness of breath, nausea, vomiting, sweating, anxiety and disorientation. Sever causes can lead to coma and death. Myocardial infraction is a common cause of death in all modern societies. Factors increasing the risk of myocardial infraction include obesity, sedentary life style, smoking and increase fat intake.

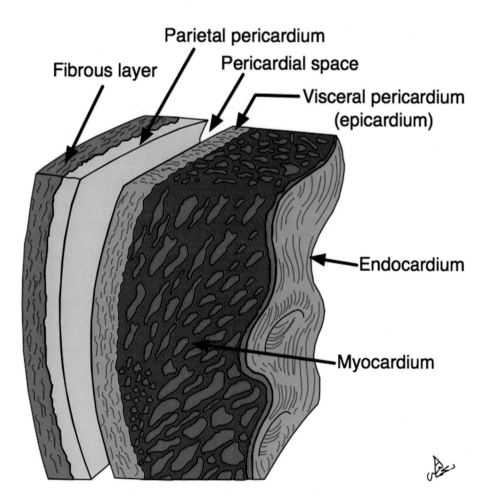

Figure 27: Illustration of the layers of the heart.

PART 6:4 FUNCTIONS

The cardiovascular system is responsible for the blood circulation. The blood circulation throughout the body is divided into systemic and pulmonary circulations. The pulmonary circulation was discovered by Alhusayn Bin Abdullah Ibn Sina (Ibn Sina), which he called the minor circulation. Together they allow the blood to bring oxygen and nutrients to the body cells and remove carbon dioxide and waste. The pulmonary circulation describes the follow of blood between the lungs and the heart only. The pulmonary arteries carry deoxygenated blood out of the right ventricle to the lungs where it becomes oxygenated. This is the only place in the body where arteries rather than veins carry deoxygenated blood. After gas exchange (carbon dioxide is exchanged for oxygen) the blood returns to the heart via the pulmonary veins. The pulmonary veins carry oxygenated blood from the lungs to the left atrium. This is the only place in the body where veins carry oxygenated blood. The systemic circulation includes the flow of blood to all parts of the body except the lungs. Oxygenated blood flows from the left atrium to the left ventricle to the aorta and is finally distributed to the body cells through many arteries. The deoxygenated blood returns to the right atrium of the heart via either the superior or inferior venae cavae (singular, vena cava).

PART 6:5 DISORDERS AND PROCEDURES

A bulge, swelling or protuberance in an artery is called an aneurysm. Angi- and vas- are the stems used to signify blood vessels. An angiogram is an X-ray film of blood vessels. Angiogenesis is the term used to describe the formation of new blood vessels, for example, in an embryo or in an adult as a result of a tumor. Veins are referred to with the terms phleob- or ven-. The term phlebectomy means the surgical removal of a vein. Arteri- is the term used for artery. Arteriosclerosis is the name for the disease characterized by hardening and narrowing of arteries due to excess fat intake and reduced physical activity. Thromb- means a blood clot. Thrombosis is the process of blood clotting. The suffix -emia refers to the blood. Bacteremia means the presence of bacteria in blood. Anemia means too few red blood cells or a condition where red blood cells are small and deficient in hemoglobin, the iron-containing red protein responsible for oxygen transport, usually a condition caused by low iron intake (iron deficiency) or due to a genetic disorder.

PART 6:6 REVIEW QUESTIONS

As a review, write the meaning for each of the following:

1. Cardio: _____

2. Angio/vaso: _____

3. Phlebo/veno: _____

4. Arterio: _____

5.-emia: _____

6.Epi: _____

7.Endo: _____

8.Peri: _____

9.Thrombo: _____

To exercise what you have learned, fill the blanks with the appropriate words:

1. The cardiovascular system consists of_____ and the_____.

2. Arteriosclerosis means _____of the_____.

3. A thrombectomy is the excision of a _____.

4. Angiospasm refers to _____.

5. _____ means too few red blood cells or a condition where red blood cells are small and deficient in _____, the iron-containing red protein responsible for oxygen transport, usually a condition caused by low iron intake (iron deficiency) or due to a genetic disorder.

6. The blood circulation throughout the body is divided into _____ and _____ circulations.

7. The walls of the heart are made of three layers. From outside to inside, these are the _____, the _____ and the _____.

8. An _____ is an X-ray film of blood vessels.

9. _____ is the term used to describe the formation of new blood vessels, for example, in an embryo or in an adult as a result of a tumor.

10. Veins are referred to with the terms _____ or _____.

11. The term _____ means the surgical removal of a vein.

12. _____ is the process of blood clotting.

13. A mobile blood clot that may occlude arteries or veins is called a _____.

14. _____ is a disease characterized by the deposition of a plaque of fatty material on the inner walls of the arteries.

15. Vasoconstruction is a condition where there is _____.

CHAPTER 7

THE RETICULOENDOTHELIAL AND IMMUNE SYSTEM

Chapter Contents

PART 7:1 INTRODUCTION

The reticuloendothelial system refers to the immune cells (leukocytes) and the structures where they are located. These structures include the liver, spleen, bone marrow, lymph nodes and lymph vessels. The immune cells include monocytes, macrophages and lymphocytes. These cells identify foreign materials, know as antigens, and destroy them. Phag- means to eat or engulf. A phagocyte is a cell that can engulf (eat) and kill invading microorganisms and foreign antigens. Phagocytosis is the ingestion of antigens (e.g., bacteria and viruses) by phagocytes.

The lymphatics, a major part of the reticuloendothelial system, consists of lymphatic vessels, lymph nodes and the lymph that runs through them. Functions of the lymphatics include fluid circulation from body tissues back to the bloodstream, absorbing fats and fat-soluble vitamins from the small intestine and also the housing of many leukocytes (mainly lymphocytes) and the filtration of lymph against pathogens and foreign bodies. The hematopoietic tissue, found in the bone marrow, contains the hematopoietic stem cells, which divide and produce the white blood cells (leukocytes), the red blood cells (erythrocytes) and the platelets (thrombocytes). In addition, the spleen and the liver are parts of the reticuloendothelial system. Both help in the detoxification and filtration of blood against toxins and pathogens.

Lymph nodes are major stations for lymphocytes and macrophages. Lymph nodes are distributed throughout the body and are linked by lymph vessels. Lymph nodes are surrounded by a fibrous capsule, which extends to the inside of the nodes as partitions called trabeculae. The interior of the lymph node is divided into the cortex in the peripheral and a medulla in the center (Figure 28). The cortex consists mainly of B lymphocytes, commonly abbreviated as B cells, arranged inside follicles. The follicles develop germinal centers when challenged with a foreign antigen. An antigen is any substance that causes an immune reaction, and normally includes viruses, bacteria, toxins, and transplanted tissues. Foreign antigens stimulate B lymphocytes to differentiate into plasma cells, which are capable of producing antibodies against the foreign antigens. Antibodies, commonly called immunoglobulins, are immune proteins capable of combating foreign antigens such as invading bacteria. An antigen-antibody reaction, also known as the immune reaction, involves binding antibodies to antigens. This reaction labels foreign antigens so that they can be recognized, and destroyed, by other cells of the immune system such as phagocytic cells. There are T lymphocytes (abbreviated as T cells), and B cells within the cortex of lymph nodes. T cells regulate the immune system by stimulating or inhibiting other immune cells. The medulla, located at the center of the lymph node, contains blood vessels and allows for exchange of immune cells with the bloodstream.

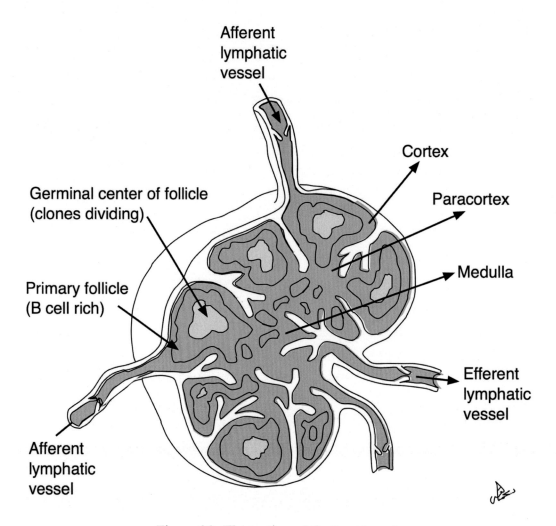

Figure 28: Illustration of the lymph node.

PART 7:2 TERMS SPECIFIC TO THE RETICULOENDOTHELIAL SYSTEM

Hema- and hemat- refer to the blood. Hematology is the science that studies the blood. Blood cells are produced by the hematopoietic stem cell found mainly in the bone marrow. An increase of the number of leukocytes over the normal limit is called leukocytosis, while a decrease in their numbers is called leukopenia. Leukocytes are divided into leukocytes that contain granules, granulocytes, and leukocytes that do not gave granules, agranulocytes (recall that the prefix a- means without).

Granulocytes, also called polymorphonuclear leukocytes because they have a nucleus with a number of lobules (poly "multiple" + morpho "shape" + nuclear "nucleus"), are characterized by the presence of differently staining granules in their cytoplasm. These granules are membrane-bound enzymes that digest phagocytosed materials (materials that are engulfed (ingested) by the cells like bacteria and viruses). There are three types of granulocytes (neutrophils, basophils and eosinophils) named according to their haematoxylin and eosin dye (H&E dye) staining characteristics. Haematoxylin, a blue dye, stains the alkaline components of the cells blue. Eosin, a red dye, stains the acidic components red. Recall that the suffix -phil denotes attraction. Thus, basophils are named because they stain dark blue, eosinophils because they stain red, and neutrophils because they stain a neutral pink (between blue and red). Eosinophils and basophils are responsible for combating multicellular parasites and play a role in allergies. Neutrophils are the most abundant type of white blood cells and are very important in most inflammatory responses.

Agranulocytes, also called mononuclear leukocytes because they have one spherical nucleus, are characterized by the apparent absence of granules in their cytoplasm. They include lymphocytes, monocytes, dendritic cells and macrophages. Lymphocytes are divided into B lymphocytes and T lymphocytes. B lymphocytes, B cells, differentiate into specialized plasma cells capable of producing antibodies. T lymphocytes, T cells, are small lymphocytes that mature in the thymus (a gland located superior to, above, the heart) as a result of exposure to the hormone thymosin, which is secreted by the thymus. T cells contribute to the immune defense by coordinating immune defenses and by killing infected cells. Dendritic cells are specialized white blood cells that patrol the body searching for foreign materials (antigens). The dendritic cells grab, swallow, and internally break apart the captured antigen. Fragments of the destroyed antigen are then moved to the surface of the cell where these fragments are displayed on tentacle-like extensions of the dendritic cell. The purpose of this display is to alert, and activate, T cells to react against this specific antigen. Macrophages (macro- "large" + -phage "eating") are large phagocytes. In addition to fighting foreign invaders via their phagocytic abilities, macrophages stimulate the action of other immune cells in a manner similar to dendritic cells. They also remove dead cells. Monocytes are small leukocytes that are found in the blood. The rapidly migrate from the blood to other tissues and differentiate to macrophages.

PART 7:3 TISSUES

The components of the reticuloendothelial system include the lymph, lymphatic vessels, lymph nodes, the liver, the spleen, the bone marrow and additional structures such as the tonsils, thymus, spleen, lacteals, Peyer's patches, vermiform appendix, and the immune cells. Lymphocytes, which are specialized immune cells, are divided into B and T cells, as mentioned above. Lymphatic circulation transports lymph from tissues throughout the body and eventually returns this fluid to the venous circulation. Lymph is a clear, watery fluid that transports waste products and proteins out of the spaces between the cells of the body tissues. It also destroys bacteria and other pathogens that are present in the tissues.

Interstitial fluid is the fluid that leaves the plasma from arterial blood to flow out of the capillaries and into the spaces between the cells. This interstitial fluid transports food, oxygen, and hormones to the cells. About 90% of this fluid is reabsorbed by the capillaries and returned to the venous circulation (reabsorbed means to be taken up again). The remaining 10% of the interstitial fluid that was not reabsorbed becomes lymph. It is transported by the lymphatic vessels and is filtered by the lymph nodes located along these vessels. Lymphatic capillaries are microscopic, blind-ended tubes. The capillary walls are only one cell in thickness. These cells separate briefly to allow lymph to enter the capillary, and the action of the cells as they close forces the lymph to flow forward. Lymph flows from the lymphatic capillaries into progressively larger lymphatic vessels, which are located deeper within the tissues. Like veins, lymphatic vessels have valves to prevent the backward flow of lymph. The larger lymphatic vessels eventually join together to form two ducts. Each duct drains a specific part of the body and returns the lymph to the venous circulation. The right lymphatic duct collects lymph from the right side of the head and neck, the upper right quadrant of the body and the right arm. The right lymphatic duct empties into the right subclavian vein (sub- "under" + clavian- "clavicle bone"), which is a major vein located under the clavicle. The thoracic duct, which is the largest lymphatic vessel in the body, collects lymph from the left side of the head and neck, the upper left quadrant of the trunk, the left arm, and the entire lower portion of the trunk and both legs. The thoracic duct empties into the left subclavian vein. Throughout the lymph vessels are located bean-shaped lymph node containing specialized lymphocytes that are capable of destroying pathogens. Unfiltered lymph flows into the nodes, and here the lymphocytes destroy harmful substances such as bacteria, viruses, and fungi. Additional structures within the node filter the lymph to remove additional impurities. After these processes are complete, the lymph leaves the node and continues its journey to again become part of the venous circulation. There are between 400 and 700 lymph nodes located along the larger lymphatic vessels, and approximately half of these nodes are in the abdomen. Most of the other nodes are positioned on the branches of the larger lymphatic vessels throughout the body. The exceptions are the three major groups of lymph nodes that are named for their locations. Cervical lymph nodes are located along the sides of the neck (cervic means neck, and -al means pertaining to). Axillary lymph nodes are located under the arms in the area known as the armpits (axill- means armpit, and -ary means pertaining to). Inguinal lymph nodes are located in the inguinal (groin) area of the lower abdomen (inguin means groin, and -al means pertaining to).

The remaining structures of this body system are made up of lymphoid tissue. The term lymphoid means pertaining to the lymphatic system or resembling lymph or lymphatic tissue. Although these structures consist of lymphoid tissue, their primary roles are in conjunction with the immune system. They include the tonsils, which are three masses of lymphoid tissue that form a protective ring around the back of the nose and the upper throat. These structures play an important role in the immune system by preventing pathogens from entering the body through the nose and mouth.

The adenoids, also known as the nasopharyngeal tonsils, are located in the nasopharynx. The palatine tonsils are located on the left and right sides of the throat in the area that is visible through the mouth. Palatine means referring to the hard and soft palates. The lingual tonsils are located at the base of the tongue (recall that lingual means pertaining to the tongue).

The thymus is located superior to (above) the heart. Although it is composed largely of lymphoid tissue, the thymus is an endocrine gland that assists the immune system. Peyer's Patches and the vermiform appendix, which consist of lymphoid tissue, protect against the entry of pathogens through the digestive system. Peyer's patches are located on the walls of the ileum. The ileum is the last section of the small intestine. The vermiform appendix hangs from the lower portion of the cecum, which is the first section of the large intestine.

The spleen is a sac-like mass of lymphoid tissue located in the left upper quadrant of the abdomen, just inferior to (below) the diaphragm and posterior to (behind) the stomach.

PART 7:4 FUNCTIONS

The primary function of the immune system is to maintain good health and to protect the body from harmful substances including: (1) pathogens, which are disease-producing microorganisms; (2) allergens, which are substances that produce allergic reactions; (3) toxins, which are poisonous or harmful substances; and (4) malignant cells, which are cancer cells.

The blood has many functions, including the transport of nutrients, oxygen and hormones to body cells and the removal of carbon dioxide and wastes. However, this exchange is not direct but is mediated through the interstitial fluid (inter "between" + stitial "to stand"). The interstitial fluid is formed from blood. Some of the interstitial fluid is drained by blood vessels, but the remaining part enters the lymphatic capillaries and is drained as lymph. Lymph nodes, distributed throughout the lymphatic capillaries, and the spleen, filter microorganisms and other foreign material from the lymph and blood, respectively. The spleen forms lymphocytes and monocytes, which are specialized white blood cells with roles in the immune system. The spleen has the hemolytic function of destroying worn-out red blood cells and releasing their hemoglobin for reuse. The spleen also stores extra erythrocytes (red blood cells) and maintains the appropriate balance between these cells and the plasma of the blood. The bone marrow also produces blood cells (white and red blood cells).

Part 7:5 Disorders and Procedures

Lymphedema, also known as swollen glands, is a common term used to describe the enlargement of lymph nodes in inflammation due to the accumulation of cells, fluids and immune components. In the word lymphedema, the prefix lymph- refers to the lymph vessels and nodes and the suffix -edema means abnormal build-up of fluid between cells (swelling of tissue). Lymphadenitis is an inflammation of the lymph nodes (recall that adeno- means gland and -itis means inflammation). Swelling and inflammation of the lymph nodes is frequently an indication of the presence of an infection. Lymphadenopathy is any disease process affecting a lymph node or nodes. A lymphangioma is a benign tumor formed by an abnormal collection of lymphatic vessels due to a congenital malformation of the lymphatic system (angi- means vessel and -oma means tumor).

Splenomegaly is an abnormal enlargement of the spleen (-megaly means abnormal enlargement). This condition can be due to bleeding caused by an injury, an infectious disease such as mononucleosis, or abnormal functioning of the immune system. Splenorrhagia is bleeding from the spleen (-rrhagia means flow).

An allergic reaction occurs when the body's immune system reacts to a harmless allergen such as pollen, food, or animal dander as if it were a dangerous invader. An allergy, also known as hypersensitivity, is an overreaction by the body to a particular antigen. The allergic response includes redness, itching, and burning. A severe systemic allergic reaction, which is also described as anaphylaxis or an anaphylactic shock, is a severe response to an allergen. Without medical aid, the patient with anaphylactic shock can die within few minutes.

Antihistamines are medications administered to relieve or prevent the symptoms of hay fever, which is a common allergy to wind-borne pollens, and other types of allergies. Antihistamines work by preventing the effects of histamine, which is a substance produced by the body that causes the itching, sneezing, runny nose, and watery eyes of an allergic reaction.

An autoimmune disorder, also known as an autoimmune disease, is any of a large group of diseases characterized by a condition in which the immune system produces antibodies against its own tissues. This abnormal functioning of the immune system appears to be genetically transmitted and predominantly occurs in women during the childbearing years. An immunodeficiency disorder occurs when the immune response is compromised (compromised means weakened, reduced, absent, or not functioning properly). The human immunodeficiency virus, commonly known as HIV, is a sexually transmitted infection in which the virus damages or kills the cells of the immune system, causing it to progressively fail, thus leaving the body at risk of developing many life-threatening opportunistic infections. This condition is called acquired immunodeficiency syndrome (AIDS). ELISA, which is the acronym for enzyme-linked immunosorbent assay, is a laboratory test used to screen for the presence of HIV antibodies. A western blot test is a blood test that produces more accurate results than the ELISA test. The western blot test is another laboratory test performed to confirm the diagnosis when the results of the ELISA test are positive. This is necessary because the ELISA test sometimes produces a false positive result in which the test erroneously indicates the presence of HIV.

Immunosuppression is treatment to repress or interfere with the ability of the immune system to respond to stimulation by antigens. An immunosuppressant is a substance that prevents or reduces the body's normal immune response. This medication is administered to prevent the rejection of donor tissue and to depress autoimmune disorders. A corticosteroid drug is a hormone-like preparation administered primarily as an anti-inflammatory and as an immunosuppressant. Vaccination, also known as immunization, is the provision of protection from communicable diseases for susceptible individuals by the administration of a vaccine to provide acquired immunity against a specific disease. A vaccine is a preparation containing an antigen, consisting of whole or partial disease-causing organisms, which have been killed or weakened.

PART 7:6 REVIEW QUESTIONS

As a review, write the meaning for each of the following:

1. Cyto: _____
2. Hema/hemato: _____
3. Spleno: _____
4. Lympho: _____
5. Phago: _____
6. AIDS: _____
7. Antihistamines: _____
8. Hypersensitivity: _____
9. Lymphadenitis: _____
10. Immunosuppression: _____
11. Immunization: _____
12. Vaccine: _____
13. Anaphylactic shock: _____
14. Malignant cells: _____
15. Antigen: _____
16. Antibody: _____
17. Toxin: _____
18. Allergens: _____
19. Pathogen: _____

To exercise what you have learned, fill the blanks with the appropriate words:

1. Cytotoxin refers to _____.
2. Hematology is the study of _____, while cytology is the study of _____.
3. A lymphocyte is a _____.
4. Splenectomy means _____.
5. Splenomegaly means _____.

List five organs of the reticuloendothelial system.

_____

_____

CHAPTER **8**

THE ENDOCRINE SYSTEM

Chapter Contents

PART 8:1 INTRODUCTION

End(o)- means within or inside and -crine means to secrete. Therefore, the endocrine system consists of secretory glands that release their secretions inside the body (into the blood stream). That is, the endocrine system consists of the glands and tissues that release signaling molecules called hormones to the blood stream. On the other hand, ex(o)- means outside, and exocrine hence means to secrete outside the blood. For example, sweat glands are exocrine glands. In addition, the glands that produce digestive juices into the stomach and small intestine are exocrine glands because they release their sections into the lumens of the stomach and intestine and not the blood stream. The pancreas is both an exocrine and an endocrine gland since it produces digestive enzymes that pour into the duodenum, the first portion of the small intestine, and hormones that are released into the blood. Endocrinology is the science that studies the endocrine system and its hormones.

Figure 29 illustrates the major glands of the body and Table 11 lists their hormones. These are: the pituitary gland, the hypothalamus, the pineal gland, the thyroid gland, the four parathyroid glands, the thymus, the pancreas, the two adrenal glands and the two gonads (ovaries or testes in females and males, respectively). These endocrine glands produce hormones. Hormones can be peptides or steroids. Peptide hormones are water-soluble and are made of amino acids. Steroid hormones are derived from cholesterol and are therefore water insoluble.

The pituitary gland, also called hypophysis, is the major body gland. A pea-sized body attached to the base of the brain, the pituitary is important in controlling growth and development and the functioning of the other endocrine glands. That is, it is physically connected to the hypothalamus. The Hypothalamus is the region of the brain that coordinates the activity of the pituitary gland, controlling body temperature, thirst, hunger, sleep and other homeostatic systems. Homeostasis, which is the process of maintaining a constant internal body environment regardless of the changing external environment (homeo "like" + stasis "standing"), is the main function of both the endocrine and nervous system.

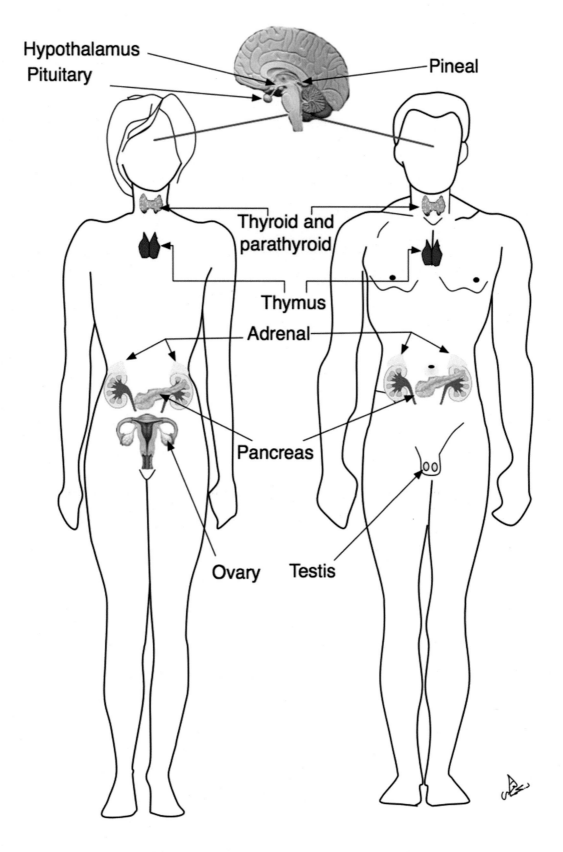

Figure 29: Illustration of the endocrine glands.

Table 11: List of hormones, their source and function

Hormone	Source	Functions
Estrogen (E)	Ovaries	Develops and maintains the female secondary sex characteristics and plays a role in the menstrual cycle and pregnancy
Follicle-stimulating hormone (FSH)	Pituitary gland	Stimulates the production of ova (eggs) and sperms in the female and male, respectively
Glucagon (GCG)	Pancreas	Increases blood glucose concentration
Growth hormone (GH)	Pituitary gland	Regulates body growth
Human chorionic gonadotropin (HCG)	Placenta	Allows the secretion of the hormones required to maintain pregnancy
Insulin	Pancreas	Allows for the transport of glucose to body cells and stimulates the conversion of excess glucose to glycogen for storage, thus lowering blood glucose concentration
Interstitial cell-stimulating hormone (ICSH)	Pituitary gland	Stimulates ovulation in the female. Stimulates the secretion of testosterone in the male
Lactogenic hormone (LTH)	Pituitary gland	Stimulates the production of breast milk and lactation
Luteinizing hormone (LH)	Pituitary gland	In the female, stimulates ovulation. In the male, stimulates testosterone secretion
Melanocyte-stimulating hormone (MSH)	Pituitary gland	Increases the production of melanin in melanocytes of the skin
Melatonin	Pineal gland	Influences the sleep-wakefulness cycles (circadian rhythm)
Norepinephrine	Adrenal medulla	Stimulates the sympathetic nervous system
Oxytocin (OXT)	Pituitary gland	Stimulates childbirth by stimulating uterine contractions during delivery. It also causes milk secretion from the mammary glands after childbirth
Parathyroid hormone (PTH)	Parathyroid glands	With calcitonin regulates calcium concentration in the blood and tissues
Progesterone	Ovaries	Completes preparation of the uterus for pregnancy
Testosterone	Testicles	Stimulates the development of male secondary sex characteristics
Thymosin	Thymus	Plays an important role in the immune system
Thyroxine (T4) and triiodothyronine (T3)	Thyroid gland	Regulates the rate of metabolism
Thyroid-stimulating hormone (TSH)	Pituitary gland	Stimulates the secretion of hormones by the thyroid gland
Adrenocorticotropic hormone	Pituitary gland	Stimulates the secretion of corticosteroids form the adrenal cortex
Vasopressin (Anti-diuretic hormone)	Pituitary gland	Released during dehydration and causes the kidneys to conserve water by producing concentrated urine
Somatostatin	Hypothalamus	Reduce the release of growth hormone

Part 8:2 Terms Specific to the Endocrine System

Polyendocrinopathy means multiple diseases in several endocrine glands (recall that poly- means many and -pathy means disease). An endocrinologist is a specialized medical professional dealing with endocrinopathies (diseases of the endocrine system). Aden- is the medical term for gland. Adenectomy means the surgical excision of a gland. Adenitis means inflammation of a gland. Adenocarcinoma and adenoma refer to cancer originating from a glandular tissue.

A suffix meaning nourishment or stimulation is -tropin (or trophin). Thus, a gonadotropin hormone is one that stimulates the functions of the gonads (the sex organs; e.g., the testes or the ovaries). Examples of gonadotropin hormones include follicle-stimulating hormone (FSH) and luteinizing hormone (LH). Hyper- and hypo- are two commonly used prefixes in endocrinology. They are used to describe the increase or decrease of the concentration of a hormone, respectively. Adrenal and adren- refer to the adrenal glands. Thus, hypoadrenalism means low adrenal gland activity. Adrenocorticotropin hormone is a hormone produced by the pituitary gland to stimulate the adrenal cortex. Hyperadrenocortism means an increase in the activity (secretions) of the adrenal cortex. The suffix -ism means condition.

Hypophys refers to the pituitary gland. Thus, hypophysitis means inflammation of the pituitary gland. Posthypophysectomy refers to the surgical removal of the posterior part of the pituitary gland. Thyr- and thyroid are the terms used to refer to the thyroid gland. Hyperthyroidism refers to an excessive activity and secretions of thyroid hormones, whereas hypothyroidism means an abnormally low production of thyroid hormones. Thyroidectomy is the surgical removal of the thyroid gland.

Part 8:3 Tissues

Secretory cells of endocrine glands release their products, hormones, into a neighboring vascularized compartment for uptake by capillaries and distribution throughout the body, rather than directly into an epithelial duct like the cells of exocrine glands. Vascularized means full with blood vessels (e.g., capillaries). Exocrine glands have a secretory portion, which contains cells specialized for secretion, and ducts, which transport the secretion of the gland to a lumen of a body organ (e.g., lumen of the intestine) or body surface. Endocrine cells typically aggregate as cords, or as follicles as in the case of the thyroid gland. Besides the specialized endocrine glands, many other organs specialized for other functions, such as the heart, thymus, gut, kidneys, testis, and ovaries, contain various endocrine cells and produce few important hormones.

Most endocrine glands are made of a parenchyma and a cortex. The parenchyma is the tissue that makes up the specialized parts of particular organs, rather than the blood vessels and connective tissue supporting structures. The cortex is the outer layer of a gland or an organ. The endocrine glands are commonly surrounded with a capsule, which sends septa into the gland. A capsule is a layer enclosing the organ. Septa, plural of septum, are partitions dividing the glands into several parts.

The thyroid gland is a highly vascular butterfly-shaped gland surrounding the anterior surface of the trachea just below the larynx. The parenchyma of the thyroid is composed of millions of rounded epithelial structures called thyroid follicles. Each follicle consists of a simple epithelium and a central lumen filled with a gelatinous substance called colloid. These epithelial cells that make the follicles are called follicular cells. Between the follicles, parafollicular cells can be found. The follicular cells produce T3 and T4 while the parafollicular cells produce calcitonin (see Table 11). The parathyroid glands are four small oval masses (nodules) located on the back of the thyroid gland. They produce parathyroid hormone (PTH). The pineal gland, also called the epiphysis cerebri, activates the rhythms of bodily activities and is located in the brain. Its secretory cells are the pinealocytes, which produce melatonin. The endocrine cells of the pancreas form clusters called the pancreatic islets (islents of Langerhans). The adrenal (suprarenal) glands are paired organs that lie at the superior poles of the kidneys. They are covered with a dense connective tissue capsule that sends thin septa into the gland. The gland consists of two concentric layers: a yellowish peripheral layer, the adrenal cortex, and a reddish-brown central layer, the adrenal medulla. The gonads – ovaries and testes – will be discussed with the female's and male's reproductive systems, respectively.

PART 8:4 FUNCTIONS

The main function of the endocrine system is to help maintain homeostasis, which is the process of maintaining a constant internal body environment regardless of the changing external environment (homeo "like" + stasis "standing"). Hormones are chemical messengers secreted by endocrine glands and have specific functions in regulating specific "target" cells and tissues. The hormones are secreted directly into the blood. Blood, or urine tests, can be used to measure hormone concentrations in the body. Table 11 above lists the most important endocrine glands, their hormones and functions.

PART 8:5 DISORDERS AND PROCEDURES

Insulin reduces the concentration of glucose sugar in blood by allowing the cells to uptake it after meals. Low insulin causes an increase in blood glucose and the appearance of sugar in urine. Gluc- and glyc- refer to glucose or any sugar, respectively. Glycosuria means the presence of sugar in urine. Hyperglycemia means high blood sugar concentration, while hypoglycemia means low blood sugar.

Acr- refers to extremity (such as the hands, feet, chin, forehead edges). Acromegaly is a disease cause by increase in growth hormone secretion leading to enlargement of the bones of the extremities.

Aden- is the stem used for gland. Adenocarcinoma is the name for cancer in glandular tissue or a cancer originating from a gland.

PART 8:6 REVIEW QUESTIONS

As a review, write the meaning for each of the following:

1. Acro: _____

2. Adeno: _____

3. Homeostasis: _____

4. Glycol: _____

To exercise what you have learned, fill the blanks with the appropriate words:

1. Hyperglycemia means _____, while hypoglycemia means _____.

2. _____ means the surgical excision of a gland.

3. _____ means inflammation of a gland

4. _____ means multiple diseases in several endocrine glands.

5. _____ means full with blood vessels (e.g., capillaries).

6. Adenocarcinoma is a cancer in _____.

7. The main function of the endocrine system is to help maintain _____, which is the process of maintaining a constant internal body environment regardless of the changing external environment.

8. The presence of sugar in urine is an abnormality known as _____.

List three glands and the hormones they produce.

_____

_____

_____

_____

_____

Name the tissue(s) that make up endocrine glands.

_____

_____

_____

_____

_____

_____

_____

CHAPTER 9

THE NERVOUS SYSTEM

Chapter Contents

PART 9:1 INTRODUCTION

The nervous system, along with the endocrine system, coordinates body functions and maintains homeostasis. Recall that homeostasis is the process of maintaining a constant internal environment regardless of the changing external environment (homeo "like" + stasis "standing"). The nervous system consists of specialized cells called neurons that transmit signals between different parts of the body and the brain. Neurons send signals as electrochemical waves traveling along thin fibers called axons, which cause chemicals called neurotransmitters to be released at cell-to-cell junctions called synapses. Electrochemical waves are a series of chemical changes that cause an electric current to develop. Neurotransmitters are chemicals that carry messages between nerve cells or between nerve cells and muscles. The electrochemical waves and the released neurotransmitters are called a nerve impulse. A cell that receives a synaptic signal may be excited or inhibited.

Anatomically, the nervous system consists of two parts: central and peripheral. The central nervous system consists of the brain and spinal cord. The peripheral nervous system consists of sensory neurons, clusters of neurons called ganglia and connecting nerves. A ganglion (plural: ganglia) is a tissue made of nerve cell bodies.

Physiologically, the nervous system is divided into somatic and autonomic nervous systems. Autonomic is an adjective meaning involuntary or unconscious. Somatic is an adjective referring to the conscious movements of the body. The autonomic system controls the viscera (internal organs of the body like the intestine). The functions of the autonomic system include controlling heart rate, respiration, salivation, digestion, perspiration, diameter of the pupils and sexual arousal. The somatic nervous system is associated with voluntary control of the body by movement of the skeletal muscles.

PART 9:2 WORD ROOTS SPECIFIC TO THE NERVOUS SYSTEM

Neur- is a stem that means nerve cell or tissue. Polyneuritis means inflammation of many nerves. Neurotoxin means a nerve poison. Neuroma is a growth of a tumor in nerve tissue. Psych- and ment- are the terms that mean mind. Psychology is the science that studies the mind.

Cerebr- and encephal- mean brain. Encephalitis means inflammation of the brain. Cerebrospinal fluid is the fluid around the brain and the spinal cord. The layers of tissues surrounding the brain and spinal cord are called the meninges. The fluid located between the spinal cord, the brain and the meninges, and within the cavities within the brain and the central canal of the spinal cord, is called the cerebrospinal fluid (CSF).

Nerve fibers are divided into efferent and afferent. Efferent means conducting outward or way from the central nervous system (the brain or spinal cord) (_E_fferent = _E_xiting the organ). Afferent means conducting toward the brain or spinal cord. Sensory neurons are activated by special stimuli and send their impulses via afferent nerves to the central nervous system. Stimuli (singular: stimulus) are anything that encourage an activity or a process to begin. Examples of stimuli that stimulate sensory neurons include: touch of skin, light falling entering the eye, and noise entering the ear. Motor neurons, located either in the central nervous system or peripheral ganglia, connect the nervous system to muscles and other effector organs via efferent nerves (an effector organ is any body part that is activated a nerve impulse).

PART 9:3 TISSUES

The nervous tissue is made of two cell types: neurons and glial cells. Glial, a Greek word meaning glue, means to provide support and nutrition to neurons. One class of glial cells, oligodendrocytes in the central nervous system and Schwann cells in the peripheral nervous system, produce fatty layers know as myelin sheets around neurons' axons to provide electric insulation allowing the electrochemical wave signals to travel quickly and strongly. In addition, they hold brain neurons in position. Certain glial cells are capable of destroying pathogens and removing dead cells and debris.

PART 9:4 FUNCTIONS

The nervous system maintains life by coordinating body functions and permitting the acquisition of food and shelter. The nervous system regulates both conscious (voluntary) and unconscious function. Regulating heart rate to provide adequate blood supply to the organs, shivering of skeletal muscles in cold weather to maintain body temperature, and fight or flight from danger are just a few of the essential functions of the nervous system. Intellect, which allows humans to create tools, equipments and ideas, is a function of the nervous system. Our understanding of the word is a consequence of the nervous system's ability to receive and interpret incoming information obtained from the many senses we have. Intelligence, the ability to memorize facts and skills, create abstract thought, understanding, communicating, reasoning, learning, retaining, planning and problem solving, is also a function of the nervous system. Psychometric testing is used to measure intelligence. The intelligence quotient (IQ) test is one of the most widely used methods for the measurement of intelligence. Other tests are used to measure certain aspects of intelligence, such as academic abilities, including GER, MCAT, GMAT and SSAT. The intelligence of humans, controlled by both environmental and genetic factors, plays a major role in determining socioeconomic status. The IQ scores of a typical population will show a normally distributed bell shaped curve (see Figure 30).

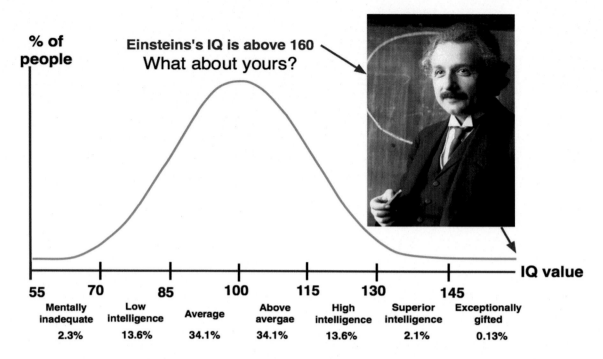

Figure 30: IQ bell curve and photograph of Albert Einstein giving a lecture in 1921.

PART 9:5 DISORDERS AND PROCEDURES

Inflammation of nerves is called neuritis. Inflammation of the layers of tissues surrounding the brain and spinal cords is called meningitis. Psychosis refers to a disorder in the state of the mind like schizophrenia. Phobia- means excessive fear. A person with hydrophobia has an excessive fear of water. Esthesia means feeling or sensation, anesthesia means without feeling or sensation, And anesthetic means a substance that reduces sensitivity to pain and feeling and may cause unconsciousness. Hyperesthesia means increased sensitivity. Pain in nerves is called neuralgia. Epilepsy is a medical disorder involving episodes of abnormal electrical discharge from the brain and characterized by periodic sudden loss or impairment of consciousness and convulsions. Convulsion, a synonym of seizure, is a violent shaking of the body or limbs caused by uncontrolled muscle contractions.

One of the most common nervous system problems is Alzheimer's disease. This disease is a disorder associated with ageing. Its symptoms include mental deterioration and loss of memory and equilibrioception (balance). In Alzheimer's the brain histology changes due to the deposition of abnormal proteins. Dementia is the general term for loss of memory and intellectual functions; a symptom associated with Alzheimer's and many other diseases and even the natural process of ageing. Another disease that is increasing in prevalence in modern societies is cerebral thrombosis. This is a very dangerous condition caused by a blood clot in a blood artery supplying the brain. This can lead to cerebral stroke, which is the death of part of the brain. Another name for cerebral thrombosis causing a stroke is cerebrovascular accident. Strokes can lead to different degrees of paralysis. Hemiplegia refers to partial paralysis of one part of the body. Paraplegia means paralysis of only the lower parts of the body: lower extremities (e.g., legs) and lower parts of the trunk. Other reasons for paralysis besides strokes are nerves injury or spinal cord damage. Surgical repair of peripheral nerves is called neuroplasty. Neuroplasty is successful for most peripheral nerves reconnected during the surgical repair of amputated parts.

PART 9:6 REVIEW QUESTIONS

As a review, write the meaning for each of the following:

1. Neuro: _____

2. Cerebro/encephalo: _____

3. Psycho/mento: _____

4. Phobia: _____

5. Esthesia: _____

6. Cerebro: _____

To exercise what you have learned, fill the blanks with the appropriate words:

1. Neuroma means _____.

2. Neurotoxin refers to _____.

3. Encephalitis is an inflammation of the _____.

4. Psychology is the science that studies the _____.

5. _____ a synonym of seizure, is a violent shaking of the body or limbs caused by uncontrolled muscle contractions.

6. A person with hemophobia (or hematophobia) has a _____ of blood.

7. _____ means paralysis of only the lower parts of the body: lower extremities (e.g., legs) and lower parts of the trunk.

8. _____ is the general term for loss of memory and intellectual functions.

9. Inflammation of nerves is called _____. Inflammation of the layers of tissues surrounding the brain and spinal cords is called _____.

10. _____ refers to a disorder in the state of the mind like schizophrenia.

11. Anesthetic is used in surgery to _____.

12. Sensory neurons are activated by special stimuli and send their impulses via _____ nerves to the central nervous system.

13. _____ means inflammation of the brain.

14. Cerebrospinal fluid is the fluid around the brain and the spinal cord.

15. The layers of tissues surrounding the brain and spinal cord are called the _____.

16. The fluid located between the spinal cord, the brain and the meninges, and within the cavities within the brain and the central canal of the spinal cord, is called the _____ _____ (CSF).

17. Neurons send signals as _____ waves traveling along thin fibers called _____, which cause chemicals called _____ to be released at cell-to-cell junctions called _____.

18. _____ (singular: stimulus) are anything that encourage an activity or a process to begin.

Is the IQ of world populations increasing or decreasing with every new generation?
(Hint: search for the Flynn effect and then refer to Lynn, R. (2008). <u>The Global Bell Curve: Race, IQ, and Inequality Worldwide</u>. Washington, USA, Washington Summit Publishers.).

CHAPTER 10

THE GENITOURINARY SYSTEM

Chapter Contents

PART 10:1 INTRODUCTION AND COMPONENTS

The genitourinary system consists of the sex and urinary organs. The urinary organs are the two kidneys, the two uteri, the urinary bladder and the urethra. The kidney is a vital organ that removes wastes, toxins, excess salts and water from the body by excreting them as urine. They contain about 2.5 million nephorns. The nephron is the basic functional unit of the kidney made of a collection of tubules and blood vessels. The urine-producing process takes place within the nephrons. The kidneys are bean shaped (e.g., have a convex and a concave surface). The concave surface is called the renal hilum and it is where the arteries, nerves, veins and the ureter enter and leave the kidney. The kidney is surrounded with a fibrous tissue called the renal capsule. The organ's parenchyma is divided into a superficial renal cortex and deep renal medulla. The medulla is organized into cone-shaped renal lobes called renal pyramids. Between the renal pyramids are projections of cortex called renal columns. The first parts of the nephrons, the renal corpuscles, are located in the cortex, while the remaining parts, the renal tubules, pass from deep in the cortex to the medulla. The tips of the pyramids, the papilla, empty urine into calyces (singular: calyx), which empty into the renal pelvis, which becomes the ureter. Inside the renal corpuscles is an extensive network of capillaries called the glomerulus. The ureters (one for each kidney) drain urine into the bladder. The bladder drains into the urethra, which opens outside the body, through the external urethra meatus. Figure 31 illustrates the structures of the renal system.

The kidneys are essential for maintaining homeostasis functions such as the regulation of water, electrolytes, acid-base balance, blood pressure and serve the function of a natural filter of the blood. By producing urine the kidneys remove wastes such as urea, ammonium, and other toxins. The kidneys also produce some hormones, including erythropoietin, calcitriol and the enzyme renin, which stimulate red blood cell production, intestinal absorption of calcium, vasoconstriction of blood vessels and the retention of water.

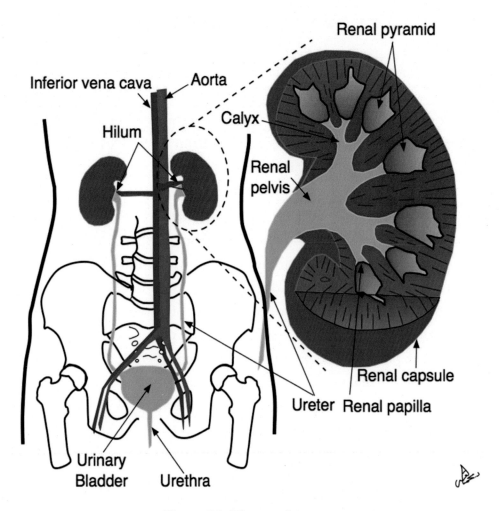

Inferior vena cava   Aorta

Hilum

Renal pyramid

Calyx

Renal
pelvis

Renal capsule

Ureter   Renal papilla

Urinary
Bladder   Urethra

Figure 31: The renal system.

The male reproductive system consists of the two testes (singular: testis) and a collection of ducts including the epididymis, ductus deferens (also called vas deferens), ejaculatory duct and urethra (Figure 32). The glands of the male's reproductive system include the seminal vesicle, prostate gland and bulbourethral gland. The penis is an accessory organ of the male's reproductive system. Sperms, also called spermatozoa, are produced in the testes, which are located in the scrotum. From there the sperms are transferred to the epididymis, which are coiled tubules located above the testes within the scrotum, where sperms complete their maturation. During ejaculation the sperms move to the vas deferens (plural: vas deferentia), which runs into the abdomen, over the top of, and behind the urinary bladder. The sperms then reach the ejaculatory ducts where the secretion of the seminal vesicles empties. Their secretions are about 60% of the total volume of semen (sperms and associated fluids) and contain mucus, amino acids and fructose. The ejaculatory ducts then empty into the urethra. The initial segment of the urethra is surrounded by the prostate gland. The prostate produces alkaline secretions to buffer the semen. The bulbourethral glands, also called Cowper's glands, are a pair of small glands located near the urethra close after the prostate. They secrete their fluids before the ejaculation of the semen to lubricate the female's reproductive canal for the insertion of the penis. The urethra, which runs from the urinary bladder through the prostate and penis, empties both urine and semen via the urinary meatus (orifice of the urethra). The penis is made of three columns of spongy erectile tissue that can be filled with blood during erection. The round head of the penis, the glans penis, is very sensitive to touch. The glans penis is covered with the foreskin, which is excised during circumcision.

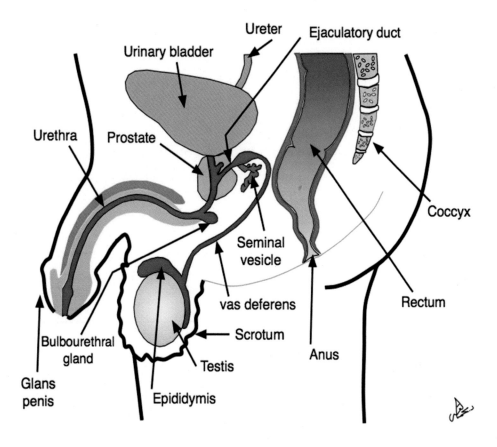

Figure 32: The male reproductive system.

The female reproductive system produces the eggs (ova; singular: ovum) and provides the site for fertilization (production of zygote through the fusion of an egg and a sperm) and embryogenesis (the formation and growth of an embryo). Ova are produced in the ovaries. Each ovum is released into the abdominal cavity near the opening of a fallopian tube (oviducts). Cilia in the fallopian tube create a current that picks the ovum. If sperms are present in the fallopian tube the ovum will be fertilized. The fertilized egg, now called a zygote, will start dividing and growing into an embryo. The embryo gets implanted in the uterus. It takes about 7 days for the zygote, or an unfertilized egg, to pass down from the fallopian tube to the uterus. The uterus has thick, muscular walls and a blood-rich lining called the endometrium. The inferior end of the uterus is called the cervix. The cervix secretes much mucus to protect the uterus and the vagina. The vagina, a canal connecting the uterus to the vulva, is about 3 inches (8 cm) long and is not only the female genital canal but also the excretory duct for the menstrual flow and the birth canal. The canal extends upward and backward. The urinary bladder is anterior to the vagina and the rectum is posterior. The vagina receives the erect penis in coitus (sexual intercourse) where spermatozoa are discharged. In a virgin, the opening of the vagina is usually partially closed by a membrane known as the hymen. Usually, the hymen breaks at first intercourse, but is can also occasionally rupture during physical exercise. The vagina is lined with a mucous membrane covering the vaginal walls, which are made of muscles and fibrous tissue. In pregnancy, changes occur in these tissues, enabling the vagina to stretch to many times its usual size allowing labor. Note that, unlike the male, the female has a separate opening for the urinary tract and reproductive system. These openings are covered with two layers of skin folds: a thin inner fold called the labia minora and a thicker outer fold called the labia majora. The labia minora contains spongy erectile tissue making it capable of changing shape when the woman is sexually aroused. At the anterior end of the labia is the clitoris. This small structure is made of erectile tissue and is rich with nerves, and is thus highly sensitive. The clitoris is the most sensitive area for female sexual stimulation. The female reproductive system is illustrated in Figure 33.

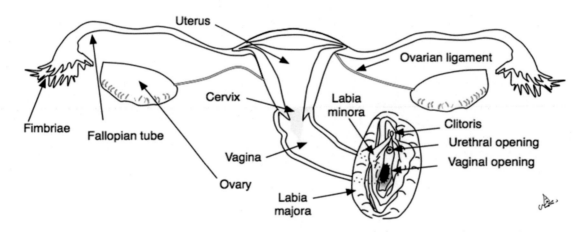

Figure 33: The female reproductive system.

PART 10:2 WORD TERMS SPECIFIC TO THE GENITOURINARY SYSTEM

Gynecology and obstetrics relate to the female's reproductive system, childbearing and birth. Orchio- means testes. Hystero- and metro- mean uterus or the womb. Hysterectomy means surgical removal of the uterus. Metrorrhagia means abnormal uterine bleeding. Oophoro- means ovary. Oophorectomy means surgical removal of the ovaries. Oophoritis means inflammation of the ovaries. Salpingo- means tube, and is the medical term used for the fallopian tubes (also called the uterine or ovarian tubes).

A very important abbreviation is UTI, which means urinary tract infection. Nephro- and rena- mean kidney. Nephritis means inflammation of the kidneys. Renal failure means breakdown of the kidneys. Uretero- means ureter. Ureteritis means inflammation of the ureter. Cyst- and -vesic- mean urinary bladder. The ureterovesical valve is the valve between the urinary bladder and the ureter. Cystitis means inflammation of the bladder. Urethr- means urethra. Urethritis is an inflammation of the urethra. Uro- and uria- are two stems for urine.

PART 10:3 FUNCTIONS

The main function of the urinary system is to filter the blood by excreting toxins and waste and regulating water and salt balance within the body. The kidneys produce the hormone erythropoietin, which stimulates erythropoiesis (production of red blood cells). In addition, the kidneys produce calcitriol, which is the hormonally active form of vitamin D. Calcitriol works to increase calcium levels in the blood by increasing its absorption from the gastrointestinal system and reducing its release with urine. The reproductive system is responsible for stimulating the secondary sexual characteristics in and the propagation of the species.

PART 10:4 DISORDERS AND PROCEDURES

Orchiopexy is the condition of the testes being fixed inside the abdomen rather than hanging normally. Orchiectomy means surgical removal of the testes. Orchidometer is the instrument used to measure testicular size. Anorchia means the absence of testes.

Hysterography means viewing the uterus using a hysteroscope. Endometritis means inflammation of the lining of the uterus. This condition can spread inside the pelvic cavity causing pelvic inflammatory disease (PID). Salpingitis means inflammation of the fallopian tube. Salping-oophorectomy means the surgical removal of uterus and ovarian tubes. Hysterosalpingography means viewing the uterus and the fallopian tubes using the hysteroscope.

Disorders of the kidneys include glomerulonephritis, which is the inflammation of the kidneys' functional units, the nephron. Blood in the urine, haematuria, and renal failure are common symptoms of glomerulonephritis. Nephrolithiasis, kidney stones, refers to the presence of mineral crystals (stones) in the renal system, which can grow large enough to block urine flow causing dysuria (painful urination). Urophobia means fear of passing urine. Bacteriuria denotes the presence of bacteria in urine due to an infection in the urinary system. Lith- means stone. Nephrolithiasis means the formation of kidney stones. Polyuria is the production of abnormally large volumes of urine. Dysuria is painful or difficult urination.

PART 10:5 REVIEW QUESTIONS

As a review, write the meaning for each of the following:
1. Nephro/reno: _____
2. Uretero: _____
3. Cysto: _____
4. Orchio: _____
5. Uro/uria: _____
6. Lith: _____
7. Hystero/metro: _____
8. Oophoro: _____
9. Salpingo: _____

To exercise what you have learned, fill the blanks with the appropriate words:
1. A person who has had his kidneys removed is said to have had a_____.
2. Inflammation of the urinary bladder is medical called _____.
3. _____ is painful or difficult urination.
4. Sperms, also called _____, are produced in the testes, which are located in the _____.
5. Urethritis is an inflammation of the_____.
6. _____ is the production of abnormally large volumes of urine.
7. Orchioectomy means _____.
8. Kidney stones are called _____.
9. Hysteroscope can be used for viewing the _____and_____.
10. Orchiopexy is the condition of the testes being fixed inside the abdomen rather than hanging normally.
11. _____ means surgical removal of the testes. _____ is the instrument used to measure testicular size.
12. _____ means the absence of testes.
13. Hysterectomy is surgical removal of the _____.
14. The glans penis is covered with the foreskin, which is excised during _____.
15. The inferior end of the uterus is called the _____.
16. The cervix secretes much _____ to protect the uterus and the vagina.
17. Oophoritis means _____.
18. The _____ system consists of the sex and urinary organs.
19. The urinary organs are the two _____, the two _____, the _____ bladder and the _____.
20. _____ means inflammation of the lining of the uterus.

21. The kidneys produce the hormone _____, which stimulates erythropoiesis (production of red blood cells). In addition, the kidneys produce _____, which is the hormonally active form of vitamin D. _____ works to increase calcium levels in the blood by increasing its absorption from the gastrointestinal system and reducing its release with urine.

22. _____ is an inflammation of the urethra.

23. _____ means inflammation of the fallopian tube.

24. _____ _____ means the surgical removal of uterus and ovarian tubes.

25. _____ means viewing the uterus and the fallopian tubes using the hysteroscope.

26. Inflammation of the uterine tubes is called _____.

Make a list of the organs that make up the female reproductive system.

_____

_____

_____

Make a list of the organs that make up the male reproductive system.

_____

_____

_____

CHAPTER 11

THE SENSORY ORGANS

Chapter Contents

PART 11:1 INTRODUCTION

In medicine and anatomy, the special senses are the senses that have specialized organs devoted for them. These include: (1) the sense of vision, which is performed by the eye; (2) hearing and balance, which is performed by the ear; (3) smelling (olfaction), which is performed by the nose; and (4) taste, which is performed by the tongue.

Other senses (general senses) like touch do not have specialized organs. Touch comes from all over the body, most noticeably from the skin, but also from the internal organs (viscera). Touch includes mechanoreception, which senses pressure, vibration and proprioception (sense of location). Other types of touch sensations include pain (nociception) and heat (thermoception). Proprioception (proprio "one's own location" + ception "sense") is the sense of the relative position of neighboring parts of the body and strength of effort being employed in movement. Another term for proprioception is kinesthesia (kin- "motion" + esthesia "sense"). The two terms are commonly used interchangeably, though kinesthesia can place a greater emphasis on motion. Nociception (noci "to hurt" + ception "sense") is the sense of potentially damaging and harmful stimuli by sending nerve signals to the spinal cord and the brain causing perception of pain. Thermoception (thermo "temperature" + ception "sense") is the sense of temperature.

PART 11:2 TERMS SPECIFIC TO THE EYE

Ophthalmo- and oculo- mean eye. Ophthalmology is the science studying the eye and its diseases. An Optometrist is the medical specialist who examines the eyes for visual defects and prescribe lenses. The human eye is an organ that reacts to light, allowing vision. The light sensitive part of the eye is the retina. In the retina, rod and cone cells allow light perception. In addition, the retina contains non-image-forming photosensitive cells, which allow adjustment to the size of the pupil, regulation of the hormone melatonin and the body clock. The pupil is the dark circular opening at the center of the iris in the eye, where light enters the eyeball to the retina. The iris is the colored part of the eye that consists of a muscular diaphragm surrounding the pupil and regulating the light entering the eyeball by expanding and contracting the pupil.

The eye is not properly a sphere; rather, it is a fused two-piece unit. The smaller frontal unit, which is more curved and called the cornea, is linked to the larger unit called the sclera. The iris – the color of the eye – and its black center, the pupil, are seen instead of the cornea due to the cornea's transparency. To see inside the eye, an ophthalmoscope is used. Thus, the eye is made of three coats. The outermost layer is made of the cornea and sclera. The middle layer consists of the choroids, ciliary body and iris. The innermost layer is the retina. Within these coats are the aqueous humor, the vitreous body and the flexible lens (see Figure 34). The eye also contains the lacrimal apparatus, which is made of the tear glands and ducts (lacrima is Latin for tears). The mucous membrane lining the eyelids is called the conjunctiva. Opto- is the stem that means vision. An optometrist is the medical specialist trained to examine vision and prescribe medical spectacles.

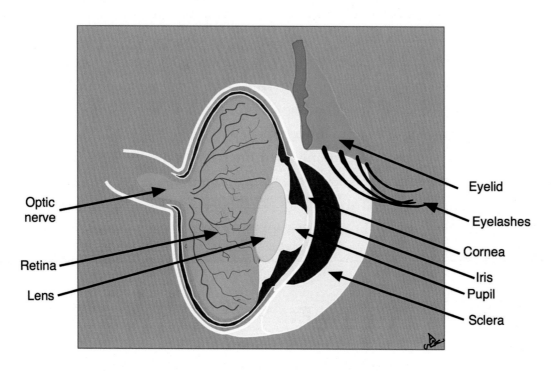

Figure 34: illustration of the eye.

PART 11:3 TERMS SPECIFIC TO HEARING AND BALANCE

Audi- means hearing or sound and oto- means ear. Otitis means inflammation of the ear. Otoplasty means surgical (plastic surgery) repair of the ear. The ear is divided into three parts: the external, middle and inner ears. The external ear is made of the auricle and the external ear canal. The auricle, also called the pinna, is made of flesh and cartilage. The external ear canal, also called the external auditory canal, extends to the tympanic membrane, the eardrum. Another name for the external auditory canal is the meatus acusticus or the acoustic meatus. In Latin, meatus means opening or passageway and acoustic means sound. The tympanic membrane is the eardrum (see Figure 35). The canal conducts sound into the middle and inner ears. The external ear is protected from infection via a wax-like substance, known as cerumen, secreted by glands in the external auditory canal. Infections of the external ear, called otitis externa, and not very common. Tympano- and myringo- refer to the eardrum. Tympanoplasty means plastic repair of the eardrum. Tympanosclerosis means abnormal hardening of the eardrum and loss of elasticity. A tympanogram is the graphic representation of change in impedance or compliance as the pressure in the ear canal is changed. Tympanometery is the measurement of the impedance of the middle ear. Myringoplasty and myringotomy are surgical repair and removal of part of the eardrum.

The tympanic membrane separates the middle and external ears. It also helps protect the middle and inner ears from injury and infection. The middle ear is sometimes called the tympanic cavity. This cavity is connected to the nasal cavity by the eustachian tube. The eustachian tube allows air pressure at both sides of the tympanic membrane to remain equal. During colds this tube sometimes gets blocked, which affects hearing and makes the patient feel as if his head is heavy. In addition, the middle ear is susceptible to infections because many organisms can travel the eustachian tube from the nasal passages. Infection of the middle ear is called otitis media. Within the middle ear three bones, called the auditory ossicles, conduct sound waves (recalling that ossi means bone, ossicle therefore means a bony part). They are the malleus (hammer), the incus (anvil) and the stapes (stirrup).

The inner ear receives sounds from the oval window (the opening of the inner ear) from the stapes and transfers it to the vestibular duct. From the vestibular duct sound travels to the membranous labyrinth (cochlea), which is a collection of canals inside the bony labyrinth. The auditory receptors, in the cochlea, finally receive the sound waves and transform them into electric signals that the brain can understand.

Equilibrioception (equilibrio "balance"), is the sense of balance, acceleration and direction of movement. It helps prevent humans from falling over when walking, standing or running. It is the result of a number of body systems working together, including the eyes (providing visual information), ears (vestibular system) and the body's sense of where it is in space (proprioception; described earlier in the introduction to this chapter). The vestibular system, the area where the semicircular canals converge (semi "similar or half") determine equilibrioception by the level of fluid in the labyrinth, which is connected to the semicircular canals. There are three semicircular canals (posterior, superior and horizontal). Movements of the fluid located inside the semicircular canals provide the brain with information about the direction and speed of motion. Each of the three semicircular canals has an enlarged area with sensory hair cells. Movement causes the fluid to move, which stimulate the hair cells.

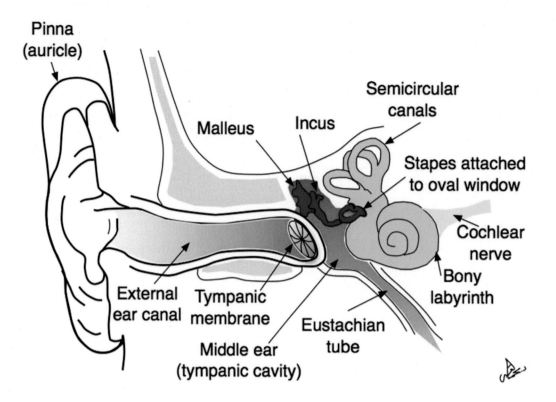

Figure 35: Illustration of the human ear.

PART 11:4 TERMS SPECIFIC TO OLFACTION AND TASTE

Olfaction, also known as olfactics, is the sense of smell. This sense is mediated by specialized sensory cells, known as olfactory receptor cells, located in the roof of the nasal cavity. Olfaction, like taste, is a form of chemoreception. Chemicals called odorants or odors activate the olfactory system. Smells are sensed by olfactory sensory neurons located in the olfactory epithelium. The olfactory sensory neurons project axons to the brain within the olfactory nerve. These axons pass to the olfactory bulb through the cribriform plate of the ethmoid bone of the skull to the brain.

In women, the sense of olfaction is strongest around the time of ovulation, significantly stronger than during other phases of the menstrual cycle and also stronger than the sense in males. Olfaction and tastes together contribute to flavor. The human tongue can distinguish only among five distinct qualities of taste while the nose can distinguish among hundreds of substances, even in minute quantities. It is during exhalation that olfaction contribution to favor occurs, in contrast to that of proper smell, which occurs during the inhalation phase.

Taste buds contain the receptors for taste. They are located on the upper surface of the tongue, lower surface of the soft plate, upper esophagus and epiglottis. The tongue, a muscular organ, is used to help chew and swallow food and talk. These taste buds are involved in detecting the five known elements of taste perception: salty, sour, bitter, sweet and umami (savoury). In 1985, at the first Umami International Symposium in Hawaii, the term umami was officially recognized as the scientific term to describe the taste of glutamates and nucleotides. It is described as a meaty taste with a long-lasting and mouthwatering sensation over the tongue.

PART 11:5 DISORDERS AND PROCEDURES

Blepharo- means eyelid. Blepharitis means inflammation of the eyelids. Kerato- means cornea. Keratitis means inflammation of the cornea. Dacryo- means tear. Dacryocystitis means inflammation of the tear sac. Myopia and hyperopia mean shortsightedness and farsightedness, respectively.

Otitis externa, otitis media and otitis interna mean inflammation of the external, middle and internal ear, respectively. Otaligia and otodynia mean pain in the ear. Vertigo means sensation of spinning due to a disorder of the inner ear. Tinnitus means sensation of noises, like ringing and buzzing, in the ears. Otoscopy means looking at the ear with an otoscope. Otorrhea means fluid discharge from the ear.

PART 11:6 REVIEW QUESTIONS

As a review, write the meaning for each of the following stems below:

1. Oto: _____
2. Tympano/myringo: _____
3. Ophthalmo/oculo: _____
4. Opto: _____
5. Blepharo: _____
6. Kerato: _____
7. Dacryo: _____

To exercise what you have learned, fill the blanks with the appropriate words:

1. The plastic repair of the ear is called _____.
2. The plastic repair of the eardrum is called _____.
3. Tympanosclerosis is the hardening of the _____.
4. Optometrist is the specialist dealing with _____ and prescribing _____.
5. _____, also known as olfactics, is the sense of smell.
6. Inflammation of the eyelids is called _____.
7. _____, _____ and _____ mean inflammation of the external, middle and internal ear, respectively.
8. The middle ear is sometimes called the tympanic cavity. This cavity is connected to the nasal cavity by the _____.
9. _____ is the science studying the eye and its diseases.
10. _____ is the sense of potentially damaging and harmful stimuli by sending nerve signals to the spinal cord and the brain causing perception of pain.
11. _____ means surgical (plastic surgery) repair of the ear.
12. The mucous membrane lining the eyelids is called the _____.
13. _____ and _____ mean shortsightedness and farsightedness, respectively.
14. Inflammation of the tear sac is called _____.

Make a list of the components that make up the human ear.

_____
_____
_____
_____
_____
_____

Make a list of the structures that make up the human eye.

_____

_____

_____

_____

_____

_____

CHAPTER 12

MICROBIOLOGY

Chapter Contents

PART 12:1 INTRODUCTION

A microorganism (micro- "small" + -organism "living creature") is a living being that is so small it can be seen only with the aid of a microscope. Contrary to popular belief, only a very limited number of microorganisms are disease causing, that is pathogens. Indeed, a human contains 10 trillion human cells and 100 trillion microorganisms. Microorganisms can have any of the following relationships with another organism: 1) symbiotic: means an interaction between a microorganism living in close physical association with the host, to the advantage of both; 2) commensal: the microorganism benefits from its host while the host derives neither benefit nor harm; 3) opportunistic: the microorganism rarely affecting humans except in unusual circumstances, typically when the immune system is weak; 4) saprophytic: the microorganism lives on dead or decaying organic matter; and 5) pathogenic: when the microorganism can cause a disease in humans. Parasite and parasitism, like pathogenic, means an organism that lives in or on another organism (its host) and benefits by deriving nutrients at the host's expense. Parasites exist in animals, plants, and microorganisms. They may live as ectoparasites (recall that ecto- is a prefix, which mean outside). Thus, ectoparasites live on the surface of the host (e.g., arthropods such as ticks, mites, lice, fleas, and many insects infesting plants and animals are ectoparasites). They can also be endoparasites (recall that endo- is a prefix, which means inside). Thus, endoparasites live in the gut or tissues of the host (e.g., many kinds of worm are endoparasites), and cause varying degrees of damage or disease to the host.

Virulence is the quality of being extremely poisonous and capable of causing disease. Thus, it is important to combat microorganisms. Destroying their ability to cause disease is called disinfection. This is usually done with a chemical disinfectant. Complete destruction (killing) of all microorganisms is called sterilization. Synonyms to the word disinfectant include: antiseptic solution, sterilizer, and decontaminant.

Microbiology is the study of microorganisms and their effects. It is divided into several branches, including virology, mycology and protozoology, and the related sciences entomology and helminthology. Protozoology, entomology and helminthology are collectively called parasitology. The definition of each of these branches of microbiology is mentioned in Table 12.

Table 12: Definition of microbiology, its brunches and related sciences

Science	Definition
Microbiology	The scientific study of microorganisms
Virology	The scientific study of viruses
Mycology	The scientific study of fungi
Protozoology	The study of protozoa, which are single-celled microscopic animals, like amoebas, flagellates, and ciliates
Entomology	The branch of science concerned with the study of arthropods
Hemlinthology	The study of parasitic worms (helminthes)
Parasitology	The branch of medicine concerned with the study of parasites

PART 12:2 TERMS SPECIFIC TO BACTERIA

Bacteria are microorganisms (singular, bacterium). Most bacteria are not harmful to humans. The full scientific name of any given bacterium species includes the genus name, followed by its species name. In this format, the genus name must be capitalized but a small letter is used for the species name, and you should either italicize both, or underline both the genus and species names. Bacteria that are pathogenic in humans include *Bacillus anthracis*, *Coxiella burnetii*, *Treponema palladium*, and *Streptococcus pneumoniae*, which cause anthrax, Q fever, syphilis and pneumonia, respectively. Based on their ability to retain a purple stain known as Gram stain, bacteria are divided into Gram-positive and Gram-negative. Gram-positive bacteria retain the stain in their thick cell wall, which is made of peptidoglycan. Peptidoglycan is made of glycan (carbohydrate) chains attached by peptide cross-bridges. The Gram-negative bacteria fail to retain the purple Gram stain because they only have a thin layer of peptidoglycan. Thus, Gram-negative bacteria appear pink and not purple.

Microorganisms, especially bacteria, are commonly named based on their shape or the disease they cause. Bacillus (plural, bacilli) means rod-shaped, and bacilli are hence rod-shaped bacteria. Tetanus, which is a sustained muscle contraction, is caused by the bacillus, *Clostridium tetani*, and is transmitted through a cut or wound. Tetanus is commonly known as lockjaw because it produces muscle spasms that are so severe a patient cannot open his or her mouth, eventually fails to breathe, and dies unless promptly treated. Spirochetes are spiral-shaped bacteria that have flexible walls and are capable of movement. Syphilis, which is a disease caused by the spirochete *Treponema pallidum*, is transmitted to humans through sexual contact. Symptoms include fever, headache, fatigue, and a characteristic skin rash. If left untreated, this infection can spread to the joints, heart, and the nervous system. Coccus (plural, cocci) is the stem meaning spherical, and thus cocci bacteria mean spherical bacteria (e.g., *Streptococcus pneumoniae*). Strept- means that the cells are arranged in chains while staph-

means that the cells are arranged in clusters. Hence, streptococci means bacteria that are spherical in shape and arranged in chains (see Figure 36). Staphylococci refers to bacteria that are spherical and arranged in grape-like clusters. Most staphylococci species are harmless and reside normally on the skin and mucous membranes of humans and other organisms; however, others are capable of producing very serious infections, especially *Staphylocuccus aureus*. Streptobacilli refers to bacteria that are rod-shaped and arranged in chains. Figure 37 illustrates bacterial shapes and provides common examples.

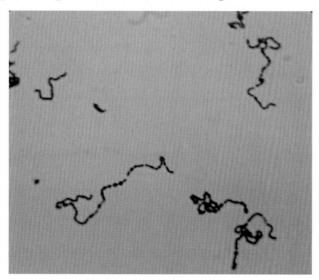

Figure 36: Microscopic view of Streptococcus pyogenes (1000 x magnification).

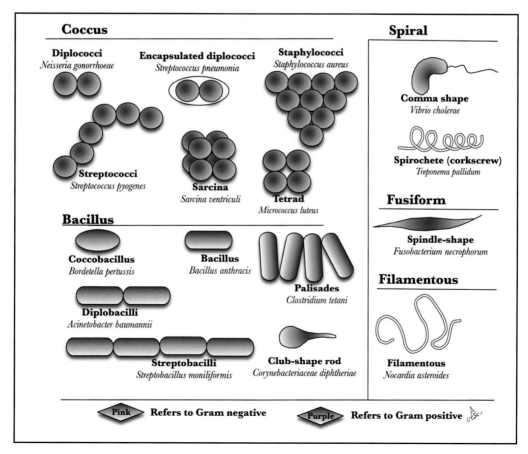

Figure 37: Illustration of bacterial shapes.

Inoculate or inoculation refers to the introduction of a microorganism into a culture or media. Inoculum refers to the material injected or placed on the media. The confluent growth area refers to the site of the inoculum where microorganisms produce thick growth of fused multiple colonies. A colony refers to a localized mass of growth of microorganisms of the same kind that originated from the same cell.

Serotype or serovar refer to distinct variations within a species of bacteria or other microorganisms based on their cell surface antigens. Determining serotypes, the process of serotyping, can be carried out by mixing the microorganism of interest with specific sera (plural form of serum) or prepared antigens. A group of serotypes with common antigens is called serogroup.

Antibiotics are medications that are capable of inhibiting growth, or killing pathogenic bacterial microorganisms (anti- "against" + bio "life" + -tic "pertaining to"). A bactericide is a substance that causes the death of bacteria (bacteri "bacteria" + -cide "causing death"). This group of antibiotics includes penicillins and cephalosporins. A bacteriostatic is an agent that slows or stops the growth of bacteria (bacteri "bacteria" + -static "not changing"). This group of antibiotics includes tetracycline, sulfonamide, and erythromycin. An antifungal (or antimycotic) is an agent that destroys or inhibits the growth of fungi. Lotrimin is an example of a topical antifungal that is applied to treat, or prevent, athlete's foot. An antiviral drug, such as acyclovir, is used to treat viral infections.

You will be able to recall that the suffix -emia means blood, and thus bacteremia and viraemia mean the presence of bacteria and viruses in the blood, respectively. Septic shock is a serious condition that occurs when an overwhelming bacterial infection affects the body. Toxins released by these pathogens can produce direct tissue damage. This damage causes vital organs (the brain, heart, kidneys, and liver) to not function properly or to fail completely. Septic shock occurs most often in the very old and the very young. It also occurs in those with underlying debilitating illnesses. Antibiotic-resistant bacteria, also known as superbugs, develop when an antibiotic fails to kill all of the bacteria it targets. When this occurs, the surviving bacteria become resistant to that particular drug. When more and more bacteria become resistant to first-line treatments, the consequences are severe, as illnesses last longer, and the risks of complications and death increase. Methicillin-resistant *Staphylococcus aureus*, commonly known as MRSA, is resistant to most antibiotics.

PART 12:3 TERMS SPECIFIC TO FUNGI

Myc- is the stem meaning fungus (plural, fungi). Mycosis means a disease caused by a fungus. Coccidioidomycosis is a fungal disease caused by the fungus *Coccidioides immitis*. Most fungi are harmless to humans, but some are pathogenic. Tinea pedis, commonly known as athlete's foot, is a fungal infection that commonly develops between the toes. Yeast is a type of fungus that is incapable of forming hyphae, which are branching filaments that make up the mycelium of a fungus. The mycelium is the vegetative part of a fungus, consisting of a network of fine filaments (hyphae). Candidiasis, commonly called thrush, is a yeast infection caused by the pathogenic yeast *Candida albicans*. Candidiasis occurs on the skin or mucous membranes. Commonly targeted locations include the vagina and the mouth.

PART 12:4 TERMS SPECIFIC TO VIRUSES

Viruses are not cells. They are not dynamic structures capable of changing or replacing its parts. A virus particle is static, having no metabolic abilities of its own. Only inside its appropriate host cell does a virus acquire a key attribute of a living system, reproduction, which then causes viral infection. One viral particle is called a virion. A virion, a virus particle, has two main parts, which are a nucleic acid core and a protein capsid (coat). Based on the nucleic acid, viruses may be either ribonucleic acid (RNA) or deoxyribonucleic acid (DNA) viruses. Some viruses are further covered with a lipid bilayer membrane called an envelope. This covers the capsid. Thus viruses can be either enveloped or naked (unenveloped). Viruses infect host cells by attaching to a receptor on the cell surface. Each virus has its specific receptor, usually a vital component of the cell surface. It is the distribution of these receptor molecules on host cells that determines the cell-preference of viruses. For example, the cold and flu virus prefers the mucus lining cells of the lungs and the airways.

PART 12:5 TERMS SPECIFIC TO PARASITES

A parasite is an organism that lives on or in a host organism and gets its food from or at the expense of its host. There are three main classes of parasites that can cause disease in humans: protozoa, helminthes (metazoan), and arthropods. Protozoa are microscopic, one-celled organisms that can be free-living or parasitic in nature. They are able to multiply in humans, which contributes to their survival and permits serious infections. Transmission of protozoa that live in a human intestine to another human typically occurs through a fecal-oral route (for example, contaminated food or water or person-to-person contact). Protozoa that live in the blood or tissue of humans are transmitted to other humans by an arthropod vector (for example, through the bite of a mosquito or sand fly).

Helminths (derived from the Greek word for worms) are large, multicellular organisms that can be visible to the unassisted eye in their adult stages. Like protozoa, helminths can be either free-living or parasitic in nature. There are three main groups of helminths that are human parasites: (1) trematodes (flukes), (2) cestodes (tapeworms) and (3) nematodes (roundworms). The adult stage of these worms can reside in the gastrointestinal tract, blood, lymphatic system or subcutaneous tissues. Alternatively, the immature (larval) states can cause disease through their infection of various body tissues. The term ectoparasites can broadly include blood-sucking arthropods such as mosquitoes, ticks, fleas, lice, and mites (because they are dependent on a blood diet from a human host for survival). Arthropods are important in causing diseases in their own right, but are even more important as vectors, or transmitters, of many different pathogens that in turn cause tremendous morbidity and mortality from the diseases they cause. Figure 38 lists the main classes of parasites

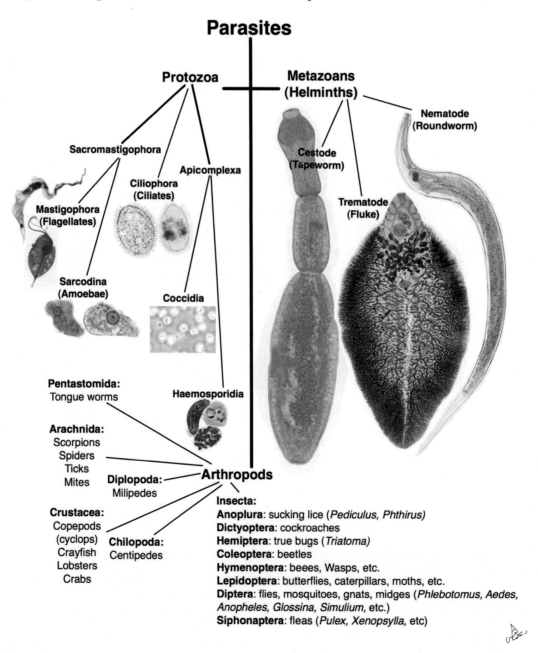

Figure 38: The classification of parasites. Note that the sizes are not to scale.

PART 12:6 REVIEW QUESTIONS

As a review, write the meaning for each of the following:

1. Microbiology: _____

2. Pathogen: _____

3. Parasite: _____

4. Helminthology: _____

5. Protozoology: _____

6. Mycosis: _____

7. Inoculation: _____

8. Streptococci: _____

9. Bacilli: _____

10. Spirochete: _____

11. Endoparasite: _____

12. Ectoparasite: _____

13. Trematodes: _____

14. Cestodes: _____

15. Nematodes: _____

16. Virus: _____

17. Arthropod: _____

18. Viraemia: _____

19. Septic shock: _____

20. Superbugs: _____

21. Confluent growth: _____

22. Bacteremia: _____

To exercise what you have learned, fill the blanks with the appropriate words:

1. There are three main groups of helminths that are human parasites: (1) _____ (_____), (2) _____ (_____) and (3) _____ (_____).

2. The term _____ can broadly include blood-sucking arthropods such as mosquitoes, ticks, fleas, lice, and mites.

3. _____ or _____ refers to the introduction of a microorganism into a culture or media. _____ refers to the material injected or placed on the media.

4. A virion, a virus particle, has two main parts, which are a nucleic acid core and a protein _____ (coat).

5. _____ means rod-shaped bacteria, which include the causative agent of tetanus, which is a sustained muscle contraction, caused by the *Clostridium tetani.*

6._____ are spiral-shaped bacteria that have flexible walls and are capable of movement.

7._____ is the stem meaning spherical, and thus _____ bacteria mean spherical bacteria (e.g., *Streptococcus pneumoniae*).

8._____ means that the cells are arranged in chains while _____ means that the cells are arranged in clusters.

9._____ mean bacteria that are spherical in shape and arranged in chains

10. _____ refer to bacteria that are spherical and arranged in grape-like clusters.

11. A microorganism is called _____ when interaction between it and the host provide advantages to both

12. Microorganisms are called _____ when the microorganism benefits from its host while the host derives neither benefit nor harm.

13. Microorganisms are called _____ when the microorganism rarely affecting humans except in unusual circumstances, typically when the immune system is weak.

14. Microorganisms are called _____ when the microorganism can cause a disease in the host.

List the names given to the different shapes of bacteria.

_____

_____

_____

_____

_____

_____

_____

_____

_____

_____

_____

_____

_____

_____

_____

_____

_____

_____

CHAPTER **13**

BIOSTATISTICS AND EPIDEMIOLOGY

Chapter Contents

PART 13:1 TERMS USED IN BIOSTATISTICS

Statistics is the science dealing with all aspects of the collection, organization, analysis, presentation and interpretation of numerical data. This includes the planning and design of surveys and experiments. A statistician is someone who conducts surveys for the collection of data and carries out the mathematical tasks for their organization, analysis, interpretation and presentation. Statistics also provides tools for the prediction and forecasting of events. The earliest writing on statistics was found in the work of the Arab scientist Al-Kindi in his book *Manuscript on Deciphering Cryptographic Messages.*

Descriptive statistics is used for summarizing or describing a collection of data. This is very useful in research when communicating the results of experiments. Inferential statistics is used to develop patterns in the data and models in a manner designed to account for randomness and uncertainty in the observation, and are used for drawing inferences about the process or population being studied. Inference is a vital element of scientific advancement, since it provides the means for drawing conclusions from data that is subject to random variation.

In statistics, it is necessary to start with a population. A population is a diverse entity, such as all persons living in a country or every atom composing a cell. Rather than collecting data from the whole population, a subset of the population, called a sample, is selected and studied using statistical analysis tools. Collecting data from the whole population is a process called a census. Obtained results include the range, mean, mode, median, variance, standard deviation and coefficient of variation.

The mean, mode and median are measures of central tendency. The median is the value that divides the data into two halves. That is, it is the numerical value separating the higher half of a sample from the lower half. The mode is the value that occurs most frequently in a data set. The sample mean ($\bar{x}$), pronounced "X bar", is the sum, Σ, of all the values divided by the number of values within the sample and is distinguished from the population mean (μ), pronounced "mu." The mean is an arithmetic value describing the central location of the data and is therefore commonly called the arithmetic average. The summation operator, Σ, is the short way to write, "take the summation of the set of numbers that follow," with the number below the Σ symbol (the subscript) referring to the first number in the data set, and the number above the Σ symbol (the superscript) is the last number. Thus the mean's equation is: $\bar{x} = \dfrac{\sum_{i=1}^{n} x_i}{n} = \dfrac{x_1 + x_2 + x_3 + ... + x_n}{n}$.

The variance for a population (δ^2), pronounced sigma square, is the measure of the degree of variation in the data from the mean. Standard deviation for a population (δ), pronounced sigma, is the square root of the variance. For a sample, the variance is S^2 and the standard deviation is S. That is, S^2 is the difference between each number and the mean divided by the number of numbers in the sample adjusted to the level of freedom ($n-1$). The

equation for calculation the variance of sample is: $S^2 = \dfrac{\sum\limits_{i=1}^{n}(x_i - \overline{x})^2}{n-1}$. The standard deviation equation for a sample is: $S = \sqrt{S^2}$.

PART 13:2 TERMS USED IN EPIDEMIOLOGY

Epidemiology (epi "upon" + demio "people" + logy "study of") is the study of the nature, causes, control, determinants and distribution of disease, disability and death in populations. That is, epidemiology is the study of the occurrence, transmission, distribution, prevention and control of disease in populations. Common terms used in epidemiology include:

1. Epidemic: a disease occurring in numbers in excess of normal expectancy.
2. Endemic: a disease or pathogen usually prevalent in a given population or geographic region at all times (from Greek: endemio "native").
3. Pandemic: a widespread epidemic distributed or occurring widely throughout a region, country, continent or globally (pan "all" + demio "people").
4. Incidence: rate of occurrence of an event, number of new cases of disease occurring over a specified period of time.
5. Prevalence: number of cases of disease occurring within a population at any given point of time.

That is, the prevalence of a disease is the number of total cases of a disease present at a particular time (numerator) in a specific population (denominator). Risk, the probability of disease, is the likelihood of an individual contracting a disease. The unit of measurement of incidence rate is cases per person-time of newly diagnosed patients. The unit of measurement of prevalence rate is the percentage of the existing population with the disease. There are two types of incidence: 1) cumulative incidence, which measures the proportion of persons who develop a disease in a given span of time; and 2) the incidence rate per 1000, which measures the rate of new disease occurrences over time and has the following equation:

Thus, epidemiology is concerned with the so-called "chain of infection," which deals with the etiological agent, source or reservoir, portal of exit, mode of transmission, portal of entry and susceptible host. The etiological agent is the cause of the disease. For example, the human immune deficiency virus is the etiological agent that causes AIDS. A reservoir is any place where the etiological agent (pathogen) resides, thrives, and reproduces without damaging it, but from which the etiological agent passes to cause disease in other organisms. Portal of exit refers to the site where the etiological agent leaves the reservoir of the patient and gains access to the outside world and to other targets. For most causes of diarrhea, for example, the portal of exit is the anus where contaminated feces leave the body to infect other victims. Portal of entry refers to the site at which the etiological agent gains entry. To illustrate, the portal of entry for most diarrheal diseases in the oral cavity and their mode of transmission is thus a fecal-oral route. A susceptible host refers to any organism (e.g., human) that can get infected by the etiological agent. A carrier, in the context of disease transmission, means an organism that carriers the etiological agent and spreads it to other organisms without usually showing the symptoms of the diseases.

Table 13: Mode of transmission of infectious diseases

Mode of Transmission	Examples
Contact Transmission	
Direct Contact: e.g., kissing, handshaking, sexual activity, blood transfusion	Gonorrhea, herpes, syphilis, HIV
Indirect Contact: e.g., spoons, coffee cups and drinking glasses, toilet seats, door handles	Common cold, influenza, mumps, measles, Q fever, pneumonia
Droplet transmission: e.g., coughing and sneezing	Streptococcal pharyngitis, pertussis, endemic syphilis
Vehicle Transmission	
Airborne: e.g., dust particles, droplets from sneezing	Chickenpox, histoplasmosis, coccidiomycosis, influenza, measles, pulmonary anthrax, tuberculosis
Foodborne: e.g., eating contaminated poultry, seafood, meat, salad	Botulism, hepatitis A and E, listeriosis, toxoplasmosis, typhoid fever, tapeworm
Waterborne: e.g., drinking, or swimming in, contaminated water	Chlera, giardia, campylobacter
Vector Transmission	
Mechanical: e.g., by getting infected from bacteria or viruses located on insect bodies (flies, cockroaches)	Trachoma, shigellosis,
Biological: e.g., by getting infected with microorganisms residing within lice, mites, mosquitoes and ticks	Lyme disease, relapsing fever, Rocky mountain spotted fever, chagas' diseases, sleeping sickness, typhus fever, yellow fever

Symptomatically, there are many forms of disease. A disease can be acute, sub-clinical, chronic, or latent. Acute describes a severe disease that quickly comes to a crisis. A sub-clinical disease is one that shows no clinical symptoms. A chronic disease is one that lasts over a long period and sometimes causes a long-term change in the body. A latent disease is one present or existing in an underdeveloped or unexpressed form (dormant) but which can develop normally under suitable conditions.

Herd immunity describes the phenomenon that occurs when the vaccination of a significant portion of a population provides protection for non-vaccinated individuals from acquiring the disease.

The incubation period is the period of time after infection is established but before the first signs of symptoms appear. It is usually dissimilar in different diseases. The epidemic curve changes depending on the incubation curve of the diseases.

Morbidity is the extent of illness, injury or disability in a defined population. Mortality is the state of being subject to death.

PART 13:3 REVIEW QUESTIONS

As a review, write the meaning for each of the following:

1. Mean (arithmetic average): _____

2. Mode: _____

3. Median: _____

4. Standard deviation: _____

5. Epidemiology: _____

6. Epidemic: _____

7. Endemic: _____

8. Pandemic: _____

9. Incidence rate: _____

To exercise what you have learned, fill the blanks with the appropriate words:

1. A place where the etiological agent of a disease resides, thrives, and reproduces without damaging it is called _____.

2. A human that can get infected by the etiological agent is said to be_____.

3._____ is used to develop patterns in the data and models for drawing inferences about the population being studied.

CHAPTER 14

SYMPTOMS, DIAGNOSIS AND SURGICAL PROCEDURES

Chapter Contents

PART 14:1 INTRODUCTION

A symptom is any indication of some disease or disorder, especially one experienced by the patient, for example, pain, dizziness, or itching. Diagnosis is the identification of an illness or disorder in a patient through an interview, physical examination and medical tests. Knowing the symptoms and diagnosis is important for the administration of the correct treatment. To reach the correct diagnosis, careful examination of the patient's symptoms and medical history is required.

Surgical procedures can have long names. Nonetheless, the meaning of most surgical procedures can usually be understood easily if their names are broken down to their basic components. For example, since hyster- means uterus and -otomy means incision, hysterotomy is an incision in the uterus. Hysterotomy is commonly used in caesarean section. Similarly, tracheotomy is the making of an incision on the anterior aspect of the neck and opening a direct airway through an incision in the trachea. It is one of the oldest described surgical procedures used to save the lives of people suffering from upper airway obstruction.

PART 14:2 TERMS SPECIFIC TO SYMPTOMS AND DIAGNOSES

Medical examination is performed during the assessment of the patient's condition in order to pave the way to arrive at a diagnosis. Vital signs are the first four key signs that are recorded. They indicate that the major body systems are functioning. These signs are temperature, heart rate, blood pressure, and respiration. The normal average body-temperature is 37°C (degrees Celsius). Hypothermia is an abnormally low body-temperature (hypo- "low" + -thermo- "temperature" + -ia "pertaining to"). Hyperthermia is an abnormally high body-temperature (fever). The pulse is the rhythmic pressure against the walls of an artery. It reflects the number of times the heart beats each minute and is recorded as beats per minute (bpm). Normally, the heart rate in adults at rest is 50-80 bpm. It is higher in children and normally each 100 to 160 in a newborn. Respiration, or respiration rate (RR), is the number of respirations per minute. One inhalation and one exhalation are counted as one respiration. In a healthy adult, the normal RR ranges from 12 to 20 respirations per minute. Blood pressure is the force exerted on the walls of arteries by the blood. This force is measured using a sphygmomanometer.

Pain is commonly considered the fifth vital sign. The suffix -algia is used to refer to pain. Dentalgia means pain in the tooth. Myalgia means pain in the muscles. Arthralgia means pain in the joints.

The suffix meaning excessive flow of discharge is -rhagia. Hemorrhage means bleeding. Menorrhagia is an abnormally heavy and prolonged menstrual period. Another suffix meaning excessive discharge of flow is -rrhea. Diarrhea is the medical term for frequent and excessive discharging of the bowels, producing abnormally thin, watery feces. Similarly, rhinorrhea and bronchorrhea mean excessive flow of nasal mucus and bronchial secretions, respectively.

The suffix meaning decrease or deficiency is -penia. Erythropenia means a decrease in the number of red blood cells. Similarly, leukopenia means a decrease in white blood cell numbers. Remember that pan is the term used for all and cyto for cells; thus, pancytopenia refers to decease in all cell types in the blood. The suffix for blood is -emia. Leukemia means the presence of an abnormal number of white blood cells. Hypoglycemia indicates a decrease in the amount of sugar in the blood.

-Spasm means involuntary contraction. The medical term myospasm then, means an involuntary contraction of the muscle. Vasospasm means involuntary contraction of the blood vessel wall. Blepharospasm, bronchospasm, and laryngospasm mean involuntary contraction of the eyelid, bronchial wall, and the larynx, respectively.

-Ectasis and -ectasia are suffixes meaning dilation or expansion. Angiectasis means abnormal dilation of a blood vessel. The suffix for prolapse or downward displacement is -ptosis. Since the stem for eyelid is blepharo, blepharoptosis means downward displacement of the eyelid. The suffix -cele means hernia, protrusion, or tumor. A gasterocele, then, is a protrusion or hernia of the stomach. The suffix for narrowing is -stenosis. Bronchostenosis refers to chronic narrowing of the bronchi.

The suffix for condition, formation of, or presence of is -asis. And since nephro- refers to the kidneys and -lithi- is the term for rocks, stones or earth, nephrolithiasis is therefore the formation of stones in the kidneys. -osis is also a suffix for condition or disease. Thrombosis is a disease caused by the formation of thrombi (blood clots). Stenosis is a disease caused by the narrowing of a vessel.

The suffix for inflammation is -itis. Encephalitis, nephritis, and enteritis mean inflammation of the brain, kidneys, and small intestine, respectively.

The suffix for softening is -malacia. Consequently, osteomalacia and chondromalacia refer to the softening of the bone and cartilage, respectively. And since the sclera is the tough, white coating of the eyeball, scleromalacia is the name given to the degenerative thinning and softening of the sclera. The suffix for hardening is -sclerosis. And since the stem for artery is arteri-, arteriosclerosis is the hardening of the arteries.

The suffix for tumor is -oma. Thus, lymphoma is a tumor originating in the lymph cells. The suffix for enlargement is -megaly. The stems for the liver and spleen, as you will recall, are hepato and spleno. Thus, hepatosplenomegaly means enlargement of both the spleen and the liver. The suffix for growth or nourishment is -trophy. The medical term for excessive growth is thus hypertrophy.

Methods used in physical examinations include palpation, percussion, and auscultation. Palpation is a medical procedure in which an organ is felt with the hands of the healthcare practitioner to determine its size, shape, firmness, and location. Percussion is a method of tapping on a body surface, to examine the underlying structure, using the middle finger of one hand, tapping on the middle finger of the other hand. Auscultation is the term for listening to the internal organs' sounds, usually using a stethoscope. Auscultation is used to examine the cardiovascular system, the respiratory system, and the gastrointestinal system.

Assessing lung sounds is an important diagnostic procedure. To auscultate lung sounds, a stethoscope is used.. There are three normal breath sounds. 1) Bronchial breath sound: This sound is loud, harsh, and high pitched. 2) Bronchovesicular breath sound: This is a blowing sound that is moderate in intensity and pitch. This sound is heard over large airways, on either side of the sternum and between scapulae. 3) Vesicular breath sound: This is a soft in quality, low-pitched sound, which is heard over the peripheral lung area and is best read at the base of the lungs. Abnormal breath sounds are called adventitious lung sounds (Table 14).

Table 14: Adventitious lung sounds

Sound	Characteristics	Disorder
Crackles	Popping, bubbling and crackling (wet sounds on inhalation)	Pulmonary edema, pulmonary fibrosis or pneumonia
Rhonchi	Rumbling sound on exhalation (continuous deep resonant sound)	Pneumonia, bronchitis, emphysema or bronchiectasis
Wheezes	High-pitched whistling sound during both inhalation and exhalation. Louder during exhalation	Asthma, anaphylactic shock, emphysema or whooping cough
Plural friction rub	Dry, grating (harsh and unpleasant) sound on both inhalation and exhalation	Pneumonia, pleural infarct, pleuritis

PART 14:3 TERMS SPECIFIC TO SURGICAL PROCEDURES

The suffix for removing or excision is -ectomy. The term salpingo means fallopian (ovarian) tube. Thus, salpingoectomy means the excision or surgical removal of the fallopian tubes. -stomy is the prefix meaning surgical creation of an artificial opening. Consequently, a colostomy is an opening made surgically into the colon. Similarly, tracheostomy, gastrostomy and nephrostomy pertain to surgical openings into the trachea, the stomach and the kidney, respectively.

The term of examination, viewing or inspection is -scopy. A bronchoscopy means examination of the inside of the bronchi. Recall that oto- refers to the ear, and thus otoscopy means examination of the inside of the ear. Similarly, colonoscopy means the examination of the colon.

-tomy is the suffix used to denote an incision or cutting into an organ. A laparotomy is thus an opening in the abdominal wall. Similarly, craniotomy is cutting (opening) into the skull (cranium) to access the brain. Thoracotomy is an incision into the chest cavity.

The suffix -pexy also mean fixation or suspension. Orchiopexy means fixation or suspending of an undescended testis (orchio- is the medical term testis). Similarly, rectopexy means fixation of the rectum with a mesh or suture. The suffix -desis means binding or fixing. Therefore, arthrodesis means the surgical binding (repair) of a dislocated joint. Ankylosis, which is a surgical procedure performed on two bones to fix a joint, such as an ankle, elbow or knee, is carried out to treat severe arthritis or a damaged joint.

The suffix for plastic surgery repair is -plasty. Tympano, as you will know by now, means eardrum. Thus, tympanoplasty means plastic repair of the eardrum. Similarly, enterocystoplasty is the surgical creation of an artificial gallbladder by isolation a segment of intestine that can be catheterized or made to drain continuously. Rhinoplasty is the term for surgical repair of the nose.

-centesis is the suffix that means puncture. Arthrocentesis means the puncture of a joint with a needle to remove fluid. Similarly, pericardiocentesis means the puncture of the pericardium and the drainage of pericardial fluid. Amniocentesis refers to the puncture of the coverings surrounding the embryo to obtain amniotic fluid for diagnosis of genetic diseases.

The medical term for suture repair is -rrhaphy. Thus, neurorrhaphy is the medical term for suture repair of a nerve. Stitching and suturing are two terms used to describe the closure of cuts and joining of body parts by a thread and a needle.

PART 14:4 REVIEW QUESTIONS

As a review, write the meaning for each of the following:

1. Diagnosis: _____
2. Therapy: _____
3. -cele: _____
4. -emia: _____
5. -ectasis: _____
6. -asis: _____
7. -itis: _____
8. -malacia: _____
9. -megaly: _____
10. -sclerosis: _____
11. -oma: _____
12. -osis: _____
13. -pathy: _____
14. -trophy: _____
15. -ptosis: _____
16. -ectomy: _____
17. -scopy: _____
18. -stomy: _____
19. -tomy: _____
20. -desis: _____
21. -pexy: _____
22. -plasty: _____
23. -centesis: _____
24. -rrhaphy: _____

To exercise what you have learned, fill the blanks with the appropriate words:

1. A gastrocele is a protrusion or _____ of the stomach.
2. Angiectasis is abnormal dilation of _____.
3. The formation of stones in the kidneys is called _____.
4. Osteomalacia is _____ of the bone.
5. Hepatomegaly means _____.
6. Hardening of the arteries is called _____.
7. A lipoma is _____.
8. Hypertrophy means _____.
9. Blepharoptosis is _____.

10. Neuropathy means _____.

11. Tonsillectomy is the surgical removal of the _____.

12. Gastroscopy means _____ of the stomach.

13. Cutting an opening through the abdominal wall is called _____.

14. Arthrodesis is the term used for _____.

15. Fixation and suspension of an undescended testis is called _____.

16. Rhinoplasty means _____.

17. Amniocentesis is the term for _____ and is used to obtain _____ fluid for the diagnosis of genetic disorders.

CHAPTER 15

MEDICAL SPECIALTIES

Chapter Contents

PART 15:1 INTRODUCTION

Specialization, to concentrate on and become expert in a particular task, is very important in all fields of life. Specialization allows for a qualitative and quantitative increase in productivity. This happens because specialization on a specific task often leads to greater skill and greater productivity on achieving this particular task than would be achieved without specialization. The fourteenth century Arab Muslim scholar, Ibn Khaldun, was one of the first to discover and emphasize the importance of the division of labor (specialization) in human activities. In his great book, *Almuqaddimah,* he stated that of necessity, a person who pursues a very specialized task will do it best. Then, through cooperation with other specialists, the requirements of a number of persons, many times greater than the specialists own number, can be satisfied. That is, through specialization and cooperation, a team of people can provide for the needs of a very large number of the population, which would not be possible if they were to work without specialization and cooperation. It is noteworthy that cooperation needs a common understanding and the ability to communicate easily. This is why every medical specialist needs to have an idea and a general understanding about all other medical specialties, to be able to cooperate effectively with their members. Nevertheless, shared principles and integration is a common theme between all specialties. That is, all specialties are intertwined. This ensures easy cooperation.

The medical field is composed of many specialties. A medical specialty is defined as any branch of medical science dealing with a specific set of diseases, or using a specific set of diagnosis methods or treatment options. For example, a surgeon uses a set of diagnostic methods and surgery options to treat diseases. He or she is not trained or able to treat diseases that require non-surgical interventions. Another example is a radiologist, who uses radiation for the diagnosis or treatment of diseases. Therefore, a radiologist cannot conduct surgical operations and a surgeon cannot use radiation to treat diseases. Nonetheless, there must be cooperation between the two. For example, many cancer patients often need both surgical operations to excise the tumor and radiation treatment (radiotherapy) to kill any remaining cancer cells. Thus, the surgeon and the radiologist work hand-in-hand for the benefit of the patient. Table 15 lists the most common medical specialties that are common worldwide.

Table 15: Common medical specialties

Subspecialty	Focus
Immunology	Concentrates on the study of immunity, including conditions such as autoimmune diseases, hypersensitivity, immune deficiency, and transplant rejection
Anaesthetic	Concentrates on anesthesia during surgical procedures and provides proper postoperative management of patients
Paediatric	Focuses on treating infants, children, and adolescents
Geriatric	Focuses on health and care of elderly people and joint replacement
Orthopedic	Focuses on treating musculoskeletal disorders
Endocrinology	Focuses on treating endocrine and hormone related diseases
Cardiothoracic surgery	Deals with diseases that need surgical attention to the thorax, such as coronary-artery bypass surgery and valve replacements
Gastroenterology	Focuses on the diagnosis and treatment of gastrointestinal disorders
Gynecology and obstetrics	Focuses on the health of the female reproductive system, pregnancy, and delivery
Internal medicine	Deals with the prevention, diagnosis, and treatment of adult diseases (especially multi-system diseases) that do not require surgery
Ophthalmology	Focuses on the health, physiology, and diseases of the eye
Vascular surgery	Focuses on the diagnosis and treatment of diseases in blood vessels
Urology	Focuses on the diagnosis and treatment of urological disorders (organs covered include the kidneys, adrenal glands, ureters, urinary bladder, urethra, testes, epididymis, prostate, vas deferens, and seminal vesicles)
Radiology	Employs radiation to treat and diagnose diseases
Psychiatry	Devoted to the study, diagnosis, and treatment of mental disorders
Rheumatology	Deals with joint, soft tissues, and vascular diseases
Plastic surgery	Concerned with the correction and restoration of form and function
Public health	Deals with preventing diseases, prolonging life, and promoting health

PART 15:2 TERMS SPECIFIC TO MEDICINE AND SURGERY

A person must graduate with a Bachelor of Medicine, Bachelor of Surgery (MBBS) to be able to practice as a general physician and a general surgeon. Graduates holding MBBS are given the courtesy title: Doctor (Dr). Nonetheless, such a graduate is more accurately called a general practitioner (GP). A general practitioner treats acute and chronic illnesses and provides preventive care and health education.

The word physician usually refers to a specialist in internal medicine or one of its many subspecialties. This meaning of physician conveys a sense of expertise in treating with drugs (medications), rather than by surgery. General practitioners specializing in internal medicine are also called internists. In contrast, a surgeon is a medical specialist concerned with the treatment of diseases and injuries by incision or manipulation (surgical operations). That is, after graduating with an MBBS, a GP can undergo postgraduate training in either internal medicine or surgery and gain a qualification in one of the many subspecialties of internal medicine or surgery. Therefore, after completing medical school, general practitioners usually further their medical education in a specific specialty of internal medicine or surgery by completing a multiple-year, residency program to become a medical specialist.

The first task carried by any medical practitioner is usually taking the medical history (also called medical case history) of the patient. The medical history consists of the answers obtained by asking specific questions of the patient himself or other people who know the patient well. The aim is to gain information useful in deriving an accurate diagnosis, to provide appropriate medical care to the patient. Following history taking, a physical examination (also called medical examination or clinical examination) is performed. While history taking is performed via asking verbal questions and collecting the answers, physical examination is the process by which the medical practitioner investigates the body of the patient for signs of disease. Methods used in physical examinations include palpation, percussion, and auscultation (see diagnosis in Chapter 14). Other specific tests may follow, which might include neurological investigation, orthopedic examination, and laboratory tests. With the results obtained from the medical history and physical examination, the medical practitioner formulates a differential diagnosis. That is, a list of potential causes of the symptoms and signs identified. Specific diagnostic tests for the suspected diseases can now be requested to attempt to provide a definite diagnosis.

After reaching a diagnosis, the medical practitioner prescribes a treatment, which can involve the administration of medications, the performance of surgeries, or both. Prescribe means advise and authorize the use of a medicine or treatment, usually by writing a prescription.

PART 15:3 TERMS SPECIFIC TO LABORATORY MEDICINE

Laboratory medicine deals with clinical specimens such as blood, urine, feces, and sputum. Tests are run on these specimens to diagnose diseases or evaluate the state of health. In addition, tests can be performed on environmental samples, medications, and foods to determine their safety. Moreover, forensic analysis of crime scene samples can be performed in the medical laboratory, to provide evidence aiding in resolving criminal investigations.

The medical laboratory is generally divided into many departments, and each department is further divided into a number of units, branches, or sections. These departments carry different tests (Table 16 list the types of specimens and tests for each laboratory medicine department). Below is a list of the most important departments and their units:

1. Microbiology: Units within this department include bacteriology, virology, parasitology, immunology, and mycology.

2. Biochemistry (clinical chemistry): This department includes enzymology, toxicology, and endocrinology.

3. Hematology: In this department, automated and manual analysis of blood cells is carried out. One of its important branches of hematology is the blood bank, which studies antigen-antibody reactions and blood types for the transfusion of blood and blood components. Transfusion is the process of receiving blood or blood components into one's circulation, intravenously. The blood bank selects donors, draws blood from them, processes the blood, and stores it to be available for transfusion.

4. Pathology: Includes units such as histopathology and cytopathology. This department studies tissues (histo- means tissue) and cells to diagnose diseases such as cancer and infection.

5. Genetics: Includes the subspecialty called cytogenetics. This department diagnoses abnormalities in chromosomes and genetic diseases. Karyotyping is one method used to study the chromosomes. Karyotyping is the examination of the appearance of chromosomes in the nucleus (recall that kary- means nucleus).

6. Reproductive biology: This department is responsible for the analysis of semen and vaginal samples.

Table 16: Specimen and test types of each laboratory medicine department

Department	Specimens	Tests
Pathology	Solid tissues (biopsies) and smears of cells	Microscopic examination to diagnose inflammation, cancer, and other diseases
Microbiology	Almost any clinical specimen, including swabs, urine, feces, blood, sputum, cerebrospinal fluid, synovial fluid, and all possibly infected tissues	Cultures to look for pathogenic microbes, biochemical tests to identify pathogens, and sensitivity tests to determine whether any isolated pathogen is resistant or sensitive to suggested antibiotics
Biochemistry	Usually receives blood and urine	Tests for lipids, sugars, enzymes, hormones, and illicit drugs
Hematology	Whole blood	Carries complete blood counts and blood films, determines blood groups, performs compatibility (cross-matching) on donors and recipients, prepares blood and blood components for transfusion
Genetics	Usually blood but can receive other tissues	Performs DNA analyses and karyotypings

PART 15:4 TERMS SPECIFIC TO NURSING

A nurse is a person trained to care for the sick. Nurses give medications and measure body temperature, blood pressure, heart rate (pulse), and respiratory rate and assist patients with basic daily needs such as bathing, toileting, and eating.

Intramuscular (IM) injection is one method a nurse must be trained to perform (Figure 39). Intramuscular injection is the introduction of a medication deep inside the muscle (recall intra- means within or inside). One area that is commonly used for this process is the mid-deltoid area (Figure 39). The deltoid is the thick, triangular muscle covering the shoulder joint, which is used for raising the arm away from the body. This area can take one milliliter of medications but not much more. A second commonly used area for intramuscular injections, which can take more than the mid-deltoid area, is the ventrogluteal area (Figure 39). This is the favorable site for adults and infants younger than twelve months because it is removed from nerves and muscular structures. A third area used for intramuscular injections is the vastus lateralis area (Figure 39). This is also a relatively safe area for injections. It is located on the anterior aspect of the thigh.

Nurses also perform intravenous infusion therapy, which is the infusion of liquid medications directly into a vein. It is commonly called a drip because it is usually applied using a drip chamber, which prevents air from entering and allows an estimation of flow rate. Thus, a nurse must be able to calculate the intravenous drip rate using the equation: (total number of milliliters) / (total number of minutes) × drip factor = drip rate. In this equation, the drip factor refers to number of drops per milliliters (gtts/ml), the total number of milliliters refers to the volume order by the physician, while the total number of minutes is the time period the physician orders the medication to be administered over.

One major cause of medical errors is the lack of understanding of the abbreviations commonly used in medicine. There are many common abbreviations that are derived from Latin, Greek, or English. Understanding these abbreviations is essential to effective communication in the medical field. Thus, every nurse must understand these common medical abbreviations, to be able to practice without endangering the health of the patients. Table 17 lists the most common medical abbreviations that are recognized worldwide by nurses, physicians, and other medical practitioners.

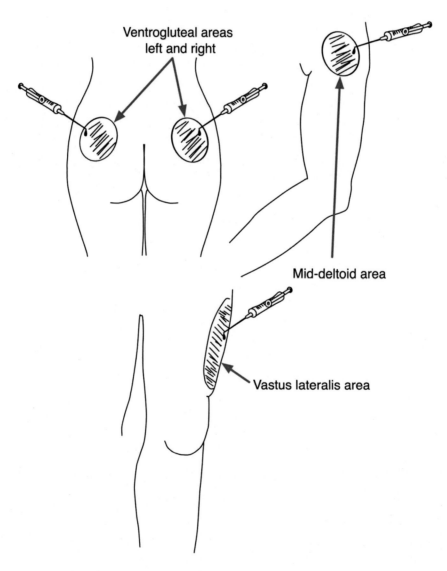

Figure 39: Intramuscular injection sites.

Table 16: Common medical abbreviations

Abbreviation	Meaning
ABG	Arterial blood gas
a.c.	Before meals
AP	Anteroposterior
ASHD	Arteriosclerotic heart disease
AV	Arteriovenous, atrioventricular
bpm	Beats per minute
CAD	Coronary artery disease
CBC	Complete blood count
CC	Chief complaint
cm	Centimeter
C&S	Culture and sensitivity
CSF	Cerebrospinal fluid
CT	Computer tomography
cu	Cubic
D/C	Discharge or discontinue
DIC	Disseminated intravascular coagulation
DSA	Digital subtraction angiography
ESR	Erythrocyte sedimentation rate
FUO	Fever of undetermined origin
g, gm	Gram
gtts	Drops
H&H	Hemoglobin and hematocrit
Hgb	Hemoglobin
Hct	Hematocrit
HS	At bed time, hours of sleep
ICS	Intercostal space
IJ	Injection
IM	Intramuscular
IN	Intranasal
IU	International unit
IV	Intravenous
Kg	Kilogram
KVO, KO	Keep vein open, keep open
KUB	Kidneys, ureters, and bladder
l	Liter
lb	Pound
IRDM	Insulin resistant diabetes mellitus

Table 17: Common medical abbreviations (*continued*)

Abbreviation	Meaning
LUQ	Left upper quadrant
m	Meter
mEq	Milliequivalent
mg	Milligram
ml	Millimeter
µl	Microliter
mm	Millimeter
NPO	Nothing by mouth
OTC	Over the counter
oz	Ounce
p.c.	After meals
PERRLA	Pupils equal, round, reactive to light and accommodation
P.O.	By mouth
prn	As needed, whenever necessary
PTCA	Percutaneous transluminal coronary angioplasty
Qh	Every hour
RLQ	Right lower quadrant
R/O	Rule out
ROM	Range of motion
RUQ	Right upper quadrant
RX	Prescription
Subq or SC	Subcutaneous
SL or S/L	Sublingual
SI	International System of Units
SOB	Short of breath, dyspnea
STD	Sexually transmitted disease
stat	Immediately
RX	Symptom
T&C	Type and cross-match
TPR	Temperature, pulse and respirations
tsp	Teaspoon
UA	Urinalysis
ung, ungt	Ointment
URI	Upper respiratory infection
UTI	Urinary tract infection
XM	Cross-match
ZSB	Zero stools since birth

PART 15:5 TERMS SPECIFIC TO RADIOLOGY

Medical radiology is the medical specialty concerned with the treatment and diagnosis of diseases by radiation. A person specialized in radiology is called a radiologist. Radiography, which is the use of X-rays, ultrasound waves, or other type of radiation to view the human body, is the main diagnostic tool used by radiologists. Radiography produces radiographs, which are images produced on sensitive plates or films by X-rays, or similar radiation. Ultrasound means sound waves (vibrations) having a frequency above the upper limit of human hearing and is used in medical imaging (e.g., ultrasound scan is commonly used to view the fetus inside the uterus during pregnancy). Tomography is the technique of displaying a representation of a cross-section through a human body, using X-rays or ultrasound waves. Computer tomography (CT scanning) is different to plain film tomography in that a computer is used to generate a three-dimensional (3 D) representation of the scanned area. Radiology is commonly used to diagnosis fractures, kidney stones, and lung diseases. Nonetheless, not all objects are visible in radiographs. For example, some kidney stones are radiolucent (e.g., uric acid stones). The term radiolucent refers to any body part that is transparent to X-rays, therefore not appearing in radiographs. On the other hand, radiopaque means not permitting the passage of X-rays or similar radiation. Thus, areas representing radiopaque parts appear white on the radiographs (e.g., bones are radiopaque).

Radiation such as X-ray can generate free radicals and create ionizing damage to living tissues and cells. Free radicals are highly reactive molecules capable of causing damage to cellular components. Free radicals and the ionizing damage can lead to mutations in DNA. Mutation, the action of mutating, is the changing of the structure of a gene (DNA), resulting in a different form that may be transmitted to subsequent daughter cells. Mutations can be silent (without any noticeable effect) or even beneficial. But, mutations caused by radiation are usually harmful and can cause cell death or cancer. Therefore, it is necessary to warn people of radiation wherever and whenever it is used. This is commonly done using the internationally recognized symbol for radiation. Figure 40 depicts this international symbol used to warn people against radiation hazards. It is worthy of note that ultrasound does not cause substantial damage (and is not associated with free radicals generation nor ionizing damage. Nonetheless, high and long exposure was found to damage the normal development of the brain in mice. Therefore, its use must be prudent and only when medically necessary and when benefits outweigh risk.

The ability of radiation to damage DNA and kill cells, increases in actively dividing cells, such as cancer cells. That is, rapidly dividing cells, such as cancer cells, are more prone to radiation damage and are more likely to be killed by it. This is why radiation is used as a cancer therapy (radiotherapy). However, because exposure to radiation is a serious hazard, all staff working in areas where ionizing radiation is a risk, needs to adhere to strict safety regulations. Protective equipment, such as a lead apron, must be worn. Moreover, staff radiation-exposure levels must be monitored using dosimeters. A lead apron is a protective garment worn over the body. In addition, thyroid shields are worn over the neck to provide protection for both the thyroid and the esophagus.

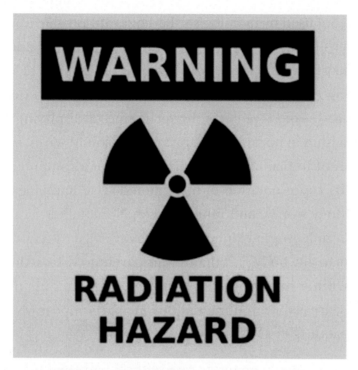

Figure 40: The radiation hazard symbol.

PART 15:6 TERMS SPECIFIC TO PHYSIOTHERAPY

Physiotherapy (also called physical therapy) is the medical specialty concerned with the treatment of diseases, injury, or deformity by physical methods such as massage, heat treatment, and exercise rather than by drugs or surgery. A medical professional specialized in physiotherapy is called physiotherapist. One of the major jobs of a physiotherapist is the promotion of mobility and functional ability. He or she is concerned with the rehabilitation of patients. Rehabilitation means to restore the patient to health or normal life by training and physical therapy after injury or disease. A physiotherapist must be well educated in human biology, anatomy, physiology, physics, clinical pathology, neuroscience, behavioral sciences, kinesiology, communication, and ethics. Kinesiology is the study of the mechanics of body movements.

Physiotherapy has many specialties, including sport physiotherapy, cardiopulmonary physiotherapy, neurologic physiotherapy, geriatric physiotherapy, orthopedic physiotherapy, and pediatric physiotherapy. These subspecialties are defined in Table 18.

Table 18: Subspecialties of physiotherapy

Subspecialty	Definition
Sport	Focuses on helping sportsmen and sportswomen to perform at their best, advises how to prevent injuries and help recover from them
Cardiopulmonary	Focuses on the assessment and treatment of acute and chronic respiratory and cardiac conditions such as postoperative rehabilitation of cardiac or pulmonary surgeries, lung inflammations, and coronary artery disease
Neurologic	Focuses on treating patients with neurological disorders such as stroke
Geriatric	Focuses on health and care of elderly people and aims to treat conditions such as osteoporosis, arthritis, Alzheimer's disease, cancer, and joint replacement
Orthopedic	Focuses on treating musculoskeletal disorders such as impaired posture, damaged muscles, and dislocated joints
Pediatric	Focuses on treating infants, children, and adolescents

Part 15:7 Terms Specific to Dentistry and Dental Hygiene

Dentistry is the specialty of medicine that involves the study, diagnosis, treatment, and prevention of diseases of the oral cavity, teeth, and the maxillofacial area. Maxillofacial means of, or relating to, the jaws and face. A dentist is the name given to a graduate from a dentistry school. He or she is qualified to treat the diseases that affect the teeth and gums, especially the repair and extraction of teeth and the insertion of artificial ones. The main two types of diseases that affect the teeth and the oral cavity are dental caries and periodontitis. Dental caries, otherwise called tooth decay or tooth cavities, is a bacterial infection that causes demineralization of the tooth enamel, dentin, and cementum (Figure 25 on page 69 shows an illustration of these structures). Periodontitis is the inflammation of the tissues around the teeth. If untreated, it often causes destruction of the gums and bones around the teeth, leading to loosening of the teeth. There are many dental subspecialties (Table 19).

Table 19: Subspecialties of dentistry

Subspecialty	Definition
Periodontics	Focuses on the supporting tissues and structures of teeth
Prosthodontics	Focuses on the rehabilitation of oral function and appearance in medical conditions associated with missing teeth, through the use of substitutes
Pediatric dentistry	Focuses on the teeth and oral cavities of children from birth to adolescence
Dental implantation	Focuses on the implantation of artificial roots, usually made of titanium, to support the restoration of missing teeth
Oral and maxillofacial surgery	Focuses on treating musculoskeletal disorders such as impaired posture, damaged muscles, and dislocated joints
Endodontics	Focuses on treating infants, children, and adolescents
Orthodontics	Focuses on the treatment of malocclusions and tooth irregularity

A dental hygienist is a medical specialist qualified to treat gum and teeth diseases and help people maintain good oral heath by educating them about how to prevent oral diseases through care of their teeth and gums. Common procedures performed by hygienists include scaling and root planing for patients with periodontitis, applying dental sealants, administration of fluoride, and providing instruction for correct oral hygiene and care. Scaling and root planing, also called conventional periodontal therapy, non-surgical periodontal therapy, deep cleaning, or dental prophylaxis, is the process of removing the etiological agents that cause periodontitis. That is, dental plaque and calculus (tartar). Figure 41 shows dental calculus on the posterior surface of the lower incisors. Dental plaque is a pale yellow film that develops on the teeth surfaces. It is mainly made of bacteria, their products, and food debris. At the beginning, dental plaque is very soft and easily removed. However, after forty-eight hours to ten days, the plaque becomes hard and transforms into calculus (Figure 41), which is very difficult to remove. The dental hygienist uses instruments such as periodontal scalers to remove the accumulated plaque and calculus. Applying dental sealants is another job performed by the dental hygienist. Dental sealants are thin plastic coatings. They are applied wherever there are grooves on the surfaces of teeth, to prevent bacteria and food debris from accumulating and causing decay. Administration of fluoride, also called fluoride therapy, is the delivery of fluoride to the teeth to prevent dental caries. Mostly fluoride is applied by using gels, toothpastes, and mouth rinses. Fluoride prevents dental caries by the formation of fluorapatite. Fluorapatite is a hard, crystalline mineral with the formula $Ca_5(PO_4)_3F$. This hard mineral enters the pores of teeth and gets deposited on their surfaces, making them harder and more resistant to decay.

Calculus (tartar)

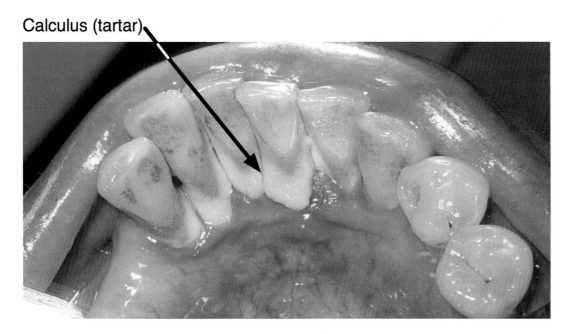

Figure 41: Calculus.

Obtained from the Department of General Dentistry, Woodhull Medical & Mental Health Center, Brooklyn, New York City, United States of America.

PART 15:8 TERMS SPECIFIC TO PUBLIC HEALTH

The focus of public health specialists is to prevent and manage diseases through the surveillance of cases and the promotion of healthy behaviors, communities, and environments. Public health can be defined as the medical specialty focused on preventing diseases, prolonging life, and enhancing health through education, promotion of healthy lifestyle, and research for disease and injury prevention. That is, public health works to prevent health problems before they occur. Indeed, many diseases are easily preventable through simple methods. For example, the simple act of hand washing with soap can prevent many infectious diseases. With the onset of antibiotics and better hygiene practices, the prevalence of infectious diseases decreased significantly in recent times, in all modern and industrialized countries. Nonetheless, chronic diseases such as cancer, heart diseases, and diabetes mellitus increased. Public health in modern countries, including Saudi Arabia, is now putting increasing attention on chronic diseases.

Public health studies the mode of transmission of infectious diseases and attempts to identify the methods necessary to prevent them. Moreover, public health deals with predisposing, protecting, precipitating, and perpetuating factors. Predisposing factors means genetic, attitudinal, personality or environmental factors that are associated with health, or lack of it, in a person or community. They include factors that render an individual vulnerable to a disease or disorder. Protecting factors are these that can protect from a disease or disorder. Precipitating factors are events that very closely precede the onset of a disease, representing a change in the situation, biologically or environmentally, and are often quite identifiable. Perpetuating factors are these factors that stop recovery from the disease and can even exacerbate the condition. After the factors associated with any disease are known, public health specialists can now work to enhance the health of individuals and communities. Top achievements in public health include:

1. Filtration and chlorination of water to prevent many water-borne diseases.
2. Fluoridation of drinking water to reduce tooth decay.
3. Recognition of tobacco use as a major health hazard.
4. Promotion of natural breast milk as the best nutrition for newborns.
5. Identifying sedentary lifestyle and high fat diet as major factors of heart diseases and strokes.
6. The promotion and the successful utilization of vaccines.

PART 15:9 TERMS SPECIFIC TO OPTOMETRY AND OPHTHALMOLOGY

Optometry is a health care profession concerned with the examination of the eyes for visual defects and the prescribing of corrective ophthalmic optics. Ophthalmic optics are any optics for the eye. This includes spectacles (glasses) and contact lenses. Ophthalmic optics are commonly referred to as optics for short. They are used to treat refractive errors. Refractive errors include myopia (nearsightedness) and hyperopia (farsightedness). That is, optometrists, also known as ophthalmic opticians, are licensed to diagnose and treat diseases of the eye through topical diagnostic and therapeutic drugs.

Ophthalmology is the medical specialty dealing with the study and treatment of diseases of the eye. A ophthalmologist is a specialist in ophthalmology. The diseases that are commonly encountered by ophthalmologists include cataracts, glaucoma, optic neuritis, vitreous hemorrhage, floaters, corneal abrasions, corneal ulcers, and photophobia. Cataracts are defined as lens opacity. That is, the lens of the eye becomes progressively opaque, resulting in poor vision. Glaucoma is progressive optic neuropathy, involving structural changes to the optic never associated with visual field changes. It is commonly associated with increased intraocular pressure. Optic neuritis means inflammation of the optic nerve. The vitreous is the clear gel that fills the posterior segment of the eye. Therefore, vitreous hemorrhage refers to bleeding inside the vitreous. This is one of the common complications of diabetes mellitus. The vitreous usually liquefies with age (syneresis). Floaters are mobile vitreous opacity casts, which are usually harmless but can sometimes cause retinal damage. They appear as gray spots or short streaks in the line of vision, which move with the eye position. Corneal ulcers are ulcers usually occurring secondary to corneal abrasion and conjunctivitis. The most common etiology of corneal ulcers is a bacterial infection. Photophobia, literally means fear of light (recall that the suffix -phobia means fear of), and is defined as light sensitivity. Causes of photophobia include iritis, meningitis, encephalitis, and glaucoma.

Part 15:10 Terms Specific to Pharmacy

Pharmacy is the science and practice of the preparation and dispensing of medicinal drugs. A pharmacist is a person who is professionally qualified to prepare and dispense medicinal drugs. Pharmacology is the branch of medicine concerned with the uses, effects, and modes of action of drugs. Abu Bakr Mohammed Ibn Yahia Ibn Zakariya Al-Razi (known in the west as Rhazes) led the field of pharmacology. Together with Abu Al-Rayhan Mohammed Ibn Ahmad Al-Birunithey (Alberonius in Latin and Al-Biruni in English), Ibn Sina (Avicenna), and Ali Ibn Al-Husain Ibn Al-Wafid (Abenguefit in Latin), Al-Birunithey succeeded in determining the specific gravity of many medications. Ibn Sina, in his famous book, *The Canon of Medicine,* described many medications and detailed characteristics and test requirements, for any medication to be accepted. *The Canon of Medicine (Al-Qanoon fi Al-Tibb)* was a standard medical text in Europe and the Islamic World until the 18th century. Ibn Al-Wafid described hundreds of medicines from various plants in his book, *Kitab al-adwiya al-mufrada* (translated into Latin as *De medicamentis simplicibus*). Abu Bakr Mohammed Ibn Yahia Ibn Zakariya Al-Razi introduced the use of ointments, mortars, flasks, and spatulas.

A pharmacist needs to know the dosage requirements, side effects, administration methods, and the pharmacodynamics of different medications. Pharmacodynamics is the branch of pharmacology concerned with the effects of drugs and the mechanisms of their actions. One important principle of pharmacy is selective toxicity.

Part 15:11 Terms Specific to Dietitians and Nutritionists

A dietician, also called a nutritionist, is a medical specialist who is an expert in nutrition or dietetics. Dietetic is the science concerned with diet and nutrition. Nutrition can be defined as the study of nutrients important to the heath of humans and the functions these nutrients perform to support the maintenance, growth, and reproduction of cells.

At the start of the twentieth century, the main aim of the science of nutrition was discovering the essential nutrients, studying deficiency state, and determining the recommended daily intake required to prevent deficiency states. An essential nutrient is any nutrient that either cannot be produced by the body at all, or cannot be produced in adequate amounts, while it is absolutely required for normal body functioning, and thus must be provided to the body from the diet. Examples of essential nutrients include vitamins, minerals, essential fatty acids, and essential amino acids. A reduction of the intake of any essential nutrient leads to health problems. This condition is called a deficiency state. For example, scurvy is a disease caused by a deficiency of vitamin C. It is characterized by swollen and bleeding gums and the opening of previously healed wounds. Scurvy particularly affected poorly nourished sailors until the end of the eighteenth century. Nonetheless, Arab sailors were immune to this condition because their diet typically contained dried dates, which contain reasonable amounts of vitamin C. The minimum daily intake, also called the recommended daily intake (RDI) is the daily intake amount of a nutrient that is considered to be adequate (sufficient) to meet the requirements of 97-98% of healthy individuals.

Nutritionists also study the digestion and absorption of foods. They determine the bioavailability of nutrients obtained from different dietary sources. Bioavailability is the proportion of a nutrient that enters the circulation (gets absorbed). It is noteworthy that the bioavailability of iron is higher from animal sources such as red meats (e.g., beef) than from plant sources (e.g., spinach). In addition, nutritionists study the net utilization of different nutrients. This concept is mainly used for proteins. The net protein utilization is a measure of food quality based on the percentage of ingested nitrogen that is retained by the body.

One area that is gaining the attention of nutritionist worldwide is antioxidants. Antioxidants are nutrients that prevent the oxidation of cellular components, such as DNA and lipids. Therefore, they are capable of preventing cancer and enhancing health. Fresh fruits and vegetables contain different varieties of antioxidants. Nonetheless, heat treatment, cooking and drying destroy most antioxidants. Thus, it is extremely important to eat uncooked and unprocessed fruits and vegetables to obtain the important health benefits of antioxidants.

PART 15:12 TERMS SPECIFIC TO PSYCHIATRY

Psychiatry is the medical specialty dedicated to the study, diagnosis, treatment and prevention of mental diseases and disorders. Mental diseases include behavioral, cognitive and perceptual abnormalities. A medical practitioner specializing in psychiatry is called a psychiatrist. Psychiatrists carry psychiatric assessments, which usually start like any typical medical assessment with taking medical history and carrying a medical examination, but they are focused on the patient's mental condition. These assessments are commonly called psychological examinations. They include neuroimaging, IQ tests (see Chapter 9), personality tests, questionnaires and mental status examinations and interviews. Neuroimaging is the use of various techniques to obtain graphical depictions of the structure and activity of the brain.

Diagnosis of mental diseases is based on criteria published in diagnostic manuals like the Diagnostic and Statistical Manual of Mental Disorders (DSM), which is published by the American Psychiatric Association, and the International Classification of Diseases (ICD), which is published by the World Health Organization. There are many drugs that are used for the treatment of many mental disorders. These are commonly called psychoactive medications.

PART 15:13 TERMS SPECIFIC TO MIDWIFERY

Midwifery is the specialty responsible for given health care to childbearing women during pregnancy, delivery and the postnatal period. Postnatal, also called postpartum, is the period following childbirth. The period before childbirth is also commonly called antenatal (recall that ante- means before; see Chapter 1 page 18). A specialist in midwifery is called a midwife. Midwives are trained to deal with low-risk pregnancy and childbirth. In addition, they are trained to recognize and manage associated conditions and disorders that can be dangerous. Obstetricians, however, are the medical specialists that are called upon to deal with illness and dangerous childbearing and childbirth situations. Therefore, midwives refer women to obstetricians when a pregnant woman requires specialist care beyond the midwives' expertise.

Midwifery services include gynecologic and family planning services, preconception care, care during pregnancy, childbirth, and the postpartum period, and care of the newborn during the first month of life. Gynecology is the branch of medicine dealing with the female reproductive system. Family planning services refer to all the services that aim to allow couples to anticipate and attain their desired number of children and control the spacing and timing between births. This is achieved through the use of contraceptives.

PART 15:14 TERMS SPECIFIC TO AMBULANCE PARAMEDICS

Emergency paramedics are healthcare specialists who work in emergency situations. They provide advanced levels of care for medical emergencies and trauma. Thus, emergency paramedics provide health care outside the hospital or clinic. They are allowed to give preliminary care and administration of emergency medications. Emergency medications include analgestics, sedatives, antiarrhythmics and antiemetics.

Common skills essential for all ambulance paramedics include: spinal injury management, fracture management, advance airway management techniques, assisting with childbirth, burn and trauma management, effective verbal and written communication skills, radio operation skills, and emergency vehicle operation.

PART 15:15 REVIEW QUESTIONS

As a review, write the meaning for each of the following:

1. Immunology: _____

2. Anaesthetic: _____

3. Paediatric: _____

4. Geriatric: _____

5. Orthopedic: _____

6. Endocrinology: _____

7. Gastroenterology: _____

8. Ophthalmology: _____

9. Radiology: _____

10. Psychiatry: _____

11. Rheumatology: _____

12. Plastic surgery: _____

13. Physician: _____

14. Internists: _____

15. Prescription: _____

16. Transfusion: _____

17. Histo-:_____

18. Karyotyping: _____

19. Ultrasound: _____

20. Tomography: _____

21. Radiolucent: _____

22. Radiopaque: _____

23. Radiograph: _____

24. Free radicals: _____

25. Radiotherapy: _____

26. Lead apron: _____

27. Rehabilitation: _____

28. Kinesiology: _____

29. Periodontitis: _____

30. Dental caries: _____

31. Periodontics: _____

32. Prosthodontics: _____

To exercise what you have learned, fill the blanks with the appropriate words:

18. A gastrocele is a protrusion or _____ of the stomach.

19. Angiectasis is abnormal dilation of _____.

20. The formation of stones in the kidneys is called _____.

21. Osteomalacia is _____ of the bone.

22. Hepatomegaly means _____.

23. Hardening of the arteries is called _____.

24. A lipoma is _____.

25. Hypertrophy means _____.

26. Blepharoptosis is _____.

27. Neuropathy means _____.

28. Tonsillectomy is the surgical removal of the _____.

29. Gastroscopy means _____ of the stomach.

30. Cutting an opening through the abdominal wall is called _____.

31. Arthrodesis is the term used for _____.

32. Fixation and suspension of an undescended testis is called _____.

33. Rhinoplasty means _____.

34. Amniocentesis is the term for _____ and is used to obtain _____ fluid for the diagnosis of genetic disorders.

Bibliography

Al-Qumber, M. and J. R. Tagg (2006). "Commensal bacilli inhibitory to mastitis pathogens isolated from the udder microbiota of healthy cows." J Appl Microbiol **101**(5): 1152-1160.

Al-Qumber, M. A. (2004). Bovine Mastitis and Human Vaginosis. Masters thesis, University of Otago, Dunedin, New Zleanad.

Allen, H. B. (2010). Dermatology Terminology. Philadelphia, USA, Springer.

Aps, J. K. and L. C. Martens (2005). "Review: The physiology of saliva and transfer of drugs into saliva." Forensic Sci Int **150**(2-3): 119-131.

Avram, M. M. (2004). "Cellulite: a review of its physiology and treatment." J Cosmet Laser Ther **6**(4): 181-185.

Barasi, M. E. (2003). Human Nutrition A Health Perspective. UK, London, Hodder Arnold.

Barber, D. (1997). "The physiology and pharmacology of pain: a review of opioids." J Perianesth Nurs **12**(2): 95-99.

Barrett, K., H. Brokks, et al. (2010). Ganong's Review of Medical Physiology. New York, USA, McGraw-Hill Medical.

Barrett, K. E. (2006). Gastrointestinal Physiology, McGraw-Hill.

Bee, D. and P. Howard (1993). "The carotid body: a review of its anatomy, physiology and clinical importance." Monaldi Arch Chest Dis **48**(1): 48-53.

Beebe, D. C. (2008). "Maintaining transparency: a review of the developmental physiology and pathophysiology of two avascular tissues." Semin Cell Dev Biol **19**(2): 125-133.

Bissada, N. K. and A. E. Finkbeiner (1980). "Smooth muscle physiology and effect of bladder and urethra muscle length/tension on response to stimulation. Part I. Review." Urology **16**(3): 323-330.

Brock, T. D. and M. T. Madigan (1988). Biology of Microorganisms. Engelwood Cliffs, Prenticc Hall.

Brodal, A. (1969). Neurological Anatomy. London, Oxford University Press.

Bukovsky, A. and M. R. Caudle (2008). "Immune physiology of the mammalian ovary - a review." Am J Reprod Immunol **59**(1): 12-26.

Burton, J. P., C. N. Chilcott, et al. (2005). "A preliminary survey of Atopobium vaginae in women attending the Dunedin gynaecology out-patients clinic: Is the contribution of the hard-to-culture microbiota overlooked in gynaecological disorders?" Aust N Z J Obstet Gynaecol **45**(5): 450-452.

Camilleri, M. and M. J. Ford (1998). "Review article: colonic sensorimotor physiology in health, and its alteration in constipation and diarrhoeal disorders." Aliment Pharmacol Ther **12**(4): 287-302.

Carey, W. D. (1977). "Colon physiology. A review." Cleve Clin Q **44**(2): 73-81.

Chambers, H. F. (2005). "Community-associated MRSA–resistance and virulence converge." N Engl J Med **352**(14): 1485-1487.

Clemente, C. D. (2011). Anatomy: A Regional Atlas of the Human Body. Philadelphia, USA, Lippincott Williams.

Coleman, P. (1979). "Antidiuretic hormone: physiology and pathophysiology - a review." J Neurosurg Nurs **11**(4): 199-204.

Compston, A. (2011). "The anatomy and physiology of cutaneous sensibility: a critical review. By FMR Walshe. Brain 1942: 65; 48-112." Brain **134**(Pt 4): 920-923.

Cook, J. C., G. R. Klinefelter, et al. (1999). "Rodent Leydig cell tumorigenesis: a review of the physiology, pathology, mechanisms, and relevance to humans." Crit Rev Toxicol **29**(2): 169-261.

Cooke, R. A. and B. Stewart (2004). Colour Atlas of Anatomical Pathology. Philadelphia, USA, Churchill Livingstone.

Culligan, K., F. H. Remzi, et al. (2012). "Review of nomenclature in colonic surgery - proposal of a standardised nomenclature based on mesocolic anatomy." Surgeon.

Cunningham, D. J. (1972). Textbook of Anatomy. London, Oxford Universty Press.

DeFriez, C. B., D. A. Morton, et al. (2011). "Orthopedic resident anatomy review course: a collaboration between anatomists and orthopedic surgeons." Anat Sci Educ **4**(5): 285-293.

den Ouden, D. T. and A. E. Meinders (2005). "Vasopressin: physiology and clinical use in patients with vasodilatory shock: a review." Neth J Med **63**(1): 4-13.

Deodhar, A. K. and R. E. Rana (1997). "Surgical physiology of wound healing: a review." J Postgrad Med **43**(2): 52-56.

Dickinson, V. A. (1978). "Maintenance of anal continence: a review of pelvic floor physiology." Gut **19**(12): 1163-1174.

Dockray, G. J. (1999). "Topical review. Gastrin and gastric epithelial physiology." J Physiol **518** (**Pt 2**): 315-324.

Eastwood, P. R., K. Takahashi, et al. (2011). "Year in review 2010: interstitial lung diseases, acute lung injury, sleep, physiology, imaging, bronchoscopic intervention and lung cancer." Respirology **16**(3): 553-563.

Edmeads, J. (1983). "The physiology of pain: a review." Prog Neuropsychopharmacol Biol Psychiatry **7**(4-6): 413-419.

Ehrlich, A. and C. L. Schroeder (2009). Medical Terminology for Health Professions. New York, USA, Delmar Cengage Learning.

Fekete, S. (1989). "Recent findings and future perspectives of digestive physiology in rabbits: a review." Acta Vet Hung **37**(3): 265-279.

Ferreira, T. S., L. D. Mangilli, et al. (2011). "Speech and myofunctional exercise physiology: a critical review of the literature." J Soc Bras Fonoaudiol **23**(3): 288-296.

Finkbeiner, W. E., P. C. Ursell, et al. (2009). Autopsy Pathology: A Manual and Atlas. Philadelphia, USA, Saunders Elsevier.

Fishburne, J. I. (1979). "Physiology and disease of the respiratory system in pregnancy. A review." J Reprod Med **22**(4): 177-189.

Flanigan, M. and S. M. Gaskell (2004). "A review of cardiac anatomy and physiology." Home Health Nurse **22**(1): 45-51.

Gavaghan, M. (1998). "Cardiac anatomy and physiology: a review." AORN J **67**(4): 802-822; quiz 824-808.

Gosmanova, E. O., V. Tangpricha, et al. (2012). "Endocrine-Metabolic Pathophysiology and Treatment Approaches Following Kidney Transplantation: a Review." Endocr Pract: 1-29.

Gruber, K. and J. Loo (2012). "Profile: German centre breathes new life into lung research." Lancet **380**(9856): 1806.

Gylys, B. A. and R. M. Masters (2010). Medical Terminology Simplified. Philadelphia, USA, F. A. Davis Company.

Halata, Z., M. Grim, et al. (2003). "Friedrich Sigmund Merkel and his "Merkel cell", morphology, development, and physiology: review and new results." Anat Rec A Discov Mol Cell Evol Biol **271**(1): 225-239.

Hawkins, R. C. (2005). "The Evidence Based Medicine approach to diagnostic testing: practicalities and limitations." Clin Biochem Rev **26**(2): 7-18.

Herlihy, B. (1983). "Physiology review. Renal physiology." Crit Care Nurse **3**(1): 101-102.

Hightower, K. R. (1985). "Cytotoxic effects of internal calcium on lens physiology: a review." Curr Eye Res **4**(4): 453-459.

Holmes, C. L., D. W. Landry, et al. (2003). "Science review: Vasopressin and the cardiovascular system part 1 - receptor physiology." Crit Care **7**(6): 427-434.

Ibn Khaldun, Rosenthal, F., Dawood, N. J. (1967). The Muqaddimah: An Introduction to History. New Jersey, USA, Princeton University Press.

Iliopoulos, C., L. Zouloumis, et al. (2010). "Physiology of bone turnover and its application in contemporary maxillofacial surgery. A review." Hippokratia **14**(4): 244-248.

Johnson, D. (1998). "Review of endocrine physiology." Semin Perioper Nurs **7**(3): 142-151.

Kantha, S. S. (1989). "A review of Nobel prizes in medicine or physiology, 1901-87." Keio J Med **38**(1): 1-12.

Kasper, D., L. Braunwald, E., Hauser, S., Longo, D., Jameson, J. L., Fauci, A. S. (2005). Harrison's Principles of Internal Medicine. New York, USA, McGraw-Hill.

Kellum, J. A. (2005). "Clinical review: reunification of acid-base physiology." Crit Care **9**(5): 500-507.

Kendrick, E. D. (1989). "Pain: a review of physiology and management options." Home Healthc Nurse **7**(6): 9-17.

Kissin, I. (2000). "Preemptive analgesia." Anesthesiology **93**(4): 1138-1143.

Kling, M. A. (2011). "A review of respiratory system anatomy, physiology, and disease in the mouse, rat, hamster, and gerbil." Vet Clin North Am Exot Anim Pract **14**(2): 287-337, vi.

Knuttinen, M. G., N. Emmanuel, et al. (2010). "Review of pharmacology and physiology in thrombolysis interventions." Semin Intervent Radiol **27**(4): 374-383.

Korner, A., S. Bluher, et al. (2005). "Obesity in childhood and adolescence: a review in the interface between adipocyte physiology and clinical challenges." Hormones (Athens) **4**(4): 189-199.

Kullander, S., G. Arvidson, et al. (1975). "A review of surfactant principles in the fetal physiology of man and animals." J Reprod Fertil Suppl(23): 659-661.

Langley, L. L. (1961). "Physiology: progress review." N Y State Dent J **27**: 5-14.

Langley-Evans, S. (2009). Nitrition: A lifespan Approach. Oxford, UK, Willey-Blackwell, A John Wiley & Sons, Ltd, publication.

Lee, K. W., K. L. Cohen, et al. (1999). "Iatrogenic vitamin D intoxication: report of a case and review of vitamin D physiology." Conn Med **63**(7): 399-403.

Linderoth, B. and R. D. Foreman (1999). "Physiology of spinal cord stimulation: review and update." Neuromodulation **2**(3): 150-164.

Ling, G. N. (1981). "Oxidative phosphorylation and mitochondrial physiology: a critical review of chemiosmotic theory, and reinterpretation by the association-induction hypothesis." Physiol Chem Phys **13**(1): 29-96.

Lynn, R. (2008). The Global Bell Curve: Race, IQ, and Inequality Worldwide. Washington, USA, Washington Summit Publishers.

Manson, P. N. (1994). "Facial bone healing and bone grafts. A review of clinical physiology." Clin Plast Surg **21**(3): 331-348.

McBain, K., I. Shrier, et al. (2012). "Prevention of sports injury I: a systematic review of applied biomechanics and physiology outcomes research." Br J Sports Med **46**(3): 169-173.

McCarthy, I. (2006). "The physiology of bone blood flow: a review." J Bone Joint Surg Am **88 Suppl 3**: 4-9.

Meldrum, B. S. (2000). "Glutamate as a neurotransmitter in the brain: review of physiology and pathology." J Nutr **130**(4S Suppl): 1007S-1015S.

Miller, J., C. Kasper, et al. (1994). "Review of muscle physiology with application to pelvic muscle exercise." Urol Nurs **14**(3): 92-97.

Mulholland, M. W. and H. T. Debas (1988). "Physiology and pathophysiology of gastrin: a review." Surgery **103**(2): 135-147.

Munarriz, R., S. W. Kim, et al. (2003). "A review of the physiology and pharmacology of peripheral (vaginal and clitoral) female genital arousal in the animal model." J Urol **170**(2 Pt 2): S40-44; discussion S44-45.

Paul, S. J. and P. Scharer (1993). "Factors in dentin bonding. Part 1: A review of the morphology and physiology of human dentin." J Esthet Dent **5**(1): 5-8.

Paul, S. J. and P. Scharer (1993). "Factors in dentin bonding. Part II: A review of the morphology and physiology of human dentin." J Esthet Dent **5**(2): 51-54.

Pena, F. J., H. Rodriguez Martinez, et al. (2009). "Mitochondria in mammalian sperm physiology and pathology: a review." Reprod Domest Anim **44**(2): 345-349.

Pollay, M. (1977). "Review of spinal fluid physiology: production and absorption in relation to pressure." Clin Neurosurg **24**: 254-269.

Quigley, S., J. Colledge, et al. (2011). "Bariatric surgery: a review of normal postoperative anatomy and complications." Clin Radiol **66**(10): 903-914.

Ramos Da Conceicao Neta, E. R., S. D. Johanningsmeier, et al. (2007). "The chemistry and physiology of sour taste - a review." J Food Sci **72**(2): R33-38.

Rao, R. S., V. Rao, et al. (2010). "Animal models in bariatric surgery - a review of the surgical techniques and postsurgical physiology." Obes Surg **20**(9): 1293-1305.

Reischman, R. R. (1988). "Review of ventilation and perfusion physiology." Crit Care Nurse **8**(7): 24-26, 28, 30.

Renn, C. L. and S. G. Dorsey (2005). "The physiology and processing of pain: a review." AACN Clin Issues **16**(3): 277-290; quiz 413-275.

Richard S. Snell, M. D., Ph.D. (1995). Clinical Anatomy for Medical Students. Toronto, Little, Brown and Company.

Salim T. S. Al-Hassani. (2012). 1001 Inventions: The Enduring Legacy of Muslim Cvilization. Random House Incorporated.

Semenza, G. L. (2007). "Vasculogenesis, angiogenesis, and arteriogenesis: mechanisms of blood vessel formation and remodeling." J Cell Biochem **102**(4): 840-847.

Spahn, D. R., B. J. Leone, et al. (1994). "Cardiovascular and coronary physiology of acute isovolemic hemodilution: a review of nonoxygen-carrying and oxygen-carrying solutions." Anesth Analg **78**(5): 1000-1021.

Stamatas, G. N., J. Nikolovski, et al. (2011). "Infant skin physiology and development during the first years of life: a review of recent findings based on in vivo studies." Int J Cosmet Sci **33**(1): 17-24.

Thomson, A. B., L. Drozdowski, et al. (2003). "Small bowel review: normal physiology, part 1." Dig Dis Sci **48**(8): 1546-1564.

Thomson, A. B., L. Drozdowski, et al. (2003). "Small bowel review: normal physiology, part 2." Dig Dis Sci **48**(8): 1565-1581.

Tipton, D. A. (1984). "A review of vision physiology." Aviat Space Environ Med **55**(2): 145-149.

Toto, K. H. (1994). "Endocrine physiology: a comprehensive review." Crit Care Nurs Clin North Am **6**(4): 637-659.

Truswell, A. S. (2003). ABC of Nutrition. London, UK, BMJ Publishing Group.

Vanderwerf, S. F. (1998). Elsevier's Medical Terminology for the Practicing Nurse. Sara Burgerhartstraat 25, Amsterdam, The Netherlands, Elsevier Science.

Vernikos, J. and V. S. Schneider (2010). "Space, gravity and the physiology of aging: parallel or convergent disciplines? A mini-review." Gerontology **56**(2): 157-166.

Viancour, T. A. (1979). "Peripheral electrosense physiology: a review of recent findings." J Physiol (Paris) **75**(4): 321-323.

Waaler, G. H. (1977). "Genetics and physiology of color vision. A review." J Oslo City Hosp **27**(11-12): 137-156.

Walter, J., D. M. Loach, et al. (2007). "D-alanyl ester depletion of teichoic acids in Lactobacillus reuteri 100-23 results in impaired colonization of the mouse gastrointestinal tract." Environ Microbiol **9**(7): 1750-1760.

Werner, J. D., G. P. Siskin, et al. (2011). "Review of venous anatomy for venographic interpretation in chronic cerebrospinal venous insufficiency." J Vasc Interv Radiol **22**(12): 1681-1690; quiz 1691.

Wexler, D. B. and T. M. Davidson (2004). "The nasal valve: a review of the anatomy, imaging, and physiology." Am J Rhinol **18**(3): 143-150.

Wilkinson, P. C. (1979). "Physiology of granulocyte locomotion and its relation to defects of chemotaxis: a review." J R Soc Med **72**(8): 606-611.

Wolfe, L. A. and T. L. Weissgerber (2003). "Clinical physiology of exercise in pregnancy: a literature review." J Obstet Gynaecol Can **25**(6): 473-483.

Woods, S. C. and R. J. Seeley (2002). "Understanding the physiology of obesity: review of recent developments in obesity research." Int J Obes Relat Metab Disord **26 Suppl** 4: S8-S10.

Yang, S. and Q. Cui (2012). "Total hip arthroplasty in developmental dysplasia of the hip: review of anatomy, techniques and outcomes." World J Orthop **3**(5): 42-48.

Zentler-Munro, P. L. and T. C. Northfield (1987). "Review: pancreatic enzyme replacement - applied physiology and pharmacology." Aliment Pharmacol Ther **1**(6): 575-591.

Zuberi, N. F. and J. H. Rizvi (2003). "Critical appraisal of endometriosis management for pain and subfertility." J Pak Med Assoc **53**(4): 152-156.

Printed in the United States
By Bookmasters